Braving The Storm: Find Hope During A Cancer Diagnosis

Braving The Storm: Find Hope During A Cancer Diagnosis

Megan Van Zyl

Braving The Storm: Find Hope During A Cancer
Diagnosis

Noble International Publishing

Copyright 2021 Megan Van Zyl

ISBN: 978-0-578-87328-2

DEDICATION

I dedicate this book to my friend, Sherry, who without you, I would not have found my passion and calling in serving cancer patients. Thank you for your life, for sharing your story with me, and for involving me in the greatest battle of your life. To some, it seems that all was lost, but I believe that you have now gained the greater part. Take care of Noble Thomas for me and I will see you soon.

ACKNOWLEDGMENTS

I want to take a moment to thank all those involved in my process of writing this book. Writing a book is an insurmountable task at times with all the other demands in personal and professional life. Thank you to those who have truly made this book manifest into reality!

Thank you first and foremost to Eugene, my husband, and Cadell Noble, my son. Thank you for supporting me through this intense process and bringing me joy and laughter!

Thank you to my mom and dad who made my life possible, supported me in every one of my life endeavors, and helped me with Cadell Noble, so that I could make the dream of this book a reality!

Thank you to my friend, Sjhira Ellzey, who inspired me, uplifted me and did all the things that only the best of friends can do!

Thank you to my friend, Kailey Oppenheim, who is my right hand woman and who helps me navigate the challenging paths of life.

Thank you to my mentor, Charles, who without your support, mentorship and encouragement, I would not have gotten this far in my path!

Thank you to my son Noble Thomas, who is praying for us from heaven and who gave me so many gifts in his short life. I can't wait to meet you one day!

Thank you to each of my cancer clients' who taught me the gift of compassion, love, and how to find beauty in the midst of the intense storms of life.

TABLE OF CONTENTS

Preface   1

Introduction   7

Section 1:
Getting Right With Me

1. A Change Of Mind: The Journey From Negativity To Positivity Is Not As Far As You Think   12

2. Releasing Regret & Shame: I Am Not My Worst Mistake   23

3. Freeing Your Mind From Imprints of Trauma   33

4. Embracing Your Eccentricity   48

5. Digging Deeper   71

Section 2:
Relationships Reflect Me: What Do You See?

1. The Broken Heart   86

2. My Soul Deserves Peace   104

3. Into Me You See   118

4. Come Out Of Hiding   133

5. The Art Of Developing True Intimacy   155

Section 3:
Unraveling the Imprint of Trauma

1. The Dream-Like State of Surviving Trauma: How to Move Past Surviving into Thriving   180

2. Mindfulness: Ending the Phantom Existence   200

3. Become a Curious Observer of Your Internal
World: Own Your Emotional Brain   218
4. Reversing the Amnesia of Trauma to Fully
Integrate Your Brain   242
5. Healing the Abandoned Heart   259

Section 4:
Wakefulness

1. Wake Up to Spiritual Reality   273
2. We All Have an Incurable Disease   289

References   314

Preface

"What is the common thread of all of my experiences, emotions and relationships that brings all of it together," my client grappled with her words to try to find a revelation to the deeper underpinnings of her diagnosis. "I'm trying to figure out what really happened to cause me to develop cancer on the emotional side. I feel that there have been so many moments of unspoken grief and pain. But what is that one thing that brings it all together?"

In a moment of clarity, I just blurted out, "Offense. Offense is when you watch what someone says and does, and you judge their motives and feel that they have done something wrong to you. Offense comes from pride and self-righteousness. Offense does not seek understanding or ask questions to figure out why someone did something, offense looks at what someone does or says at face value. The person who becomes offended decides what the other person did was very wrong and not something that they would ever do. Offense separates relationships, making it very difficult to forgive and build long-lasting, meaningful relationships with friends and family members."

1

My client gasped out in surprise, "That's it. Many people have offended me in my life. That's the common thread. Offense. Wow. I never knew."

Months before this moment, my client had been in the hospital needing tubes to help her lungs drain fluid out as one of the many side effects of her medication. It was a miracle that we had even gotten to this point in the conversation as our sessions were delayed by hospital visits and a long list of life-threatening side effects.

I will never forget when my client emailed me the following email, "My CT scan showed scar tissue on my lungs and that my bones are healing." Joyful laughter bubbled from my mouth as I took a breath and seared this moment into my memory with deep gratitude. This is why I do what I do. Moments like this make it all worth it, I thought to myself. I will never stop working with cancer patients to pursue spontaneous remission (remission that is not expected by their oncologist).

Spontaneous remission from cancer doesn't occur all the time in my practice, but when it does, it is the most precious and valuable moment that I can measure in my life. It is worth pursuing in every case of an incurable cancer diagnosis.

Every time I work with someone diagnosed with cancer, I learn something new. I change my perspective on what cancer is and how it manifests through a person's life. What is the common thread? Trying to find the common thread of emotional patterns, relational patterns and experiences of trauma is not always as simple and revelatory as it was with this client. Some of my clients have layers upon layers of painful, traumatic memories that are woven into a never-ending book that is overwhelmingly complicated.

I write this book for many reasons. But the first reason is to develop a guidebook; a glimpse into the common threads of spontaneous remission, which helps an overwhelmingly complicated situation become less complicated and the path of spontaneous remission clearer. My goal is to help those with an incurable cancer diagnosis to find the clarity needed to move forward in a meaningful way. What can happen is simple: my clients can become so obsessively focused on eating enough broccoli that they overlook the big picture and common threads of unresolved emotional and relational conflict. Thus, the thought patterns and emotional patterns of anger, resentment, hate, pain, grief and trauma pulse throughout the body, day in and day out, as we try to eat enough foods with nutritional value to fight against the progression of cancer within our body.

But we lose the big picture: the complexity of the human mind and soul and what it truly takes to put cancer in its place. We need to magnify our true identity, establish meaningful connection with others, and ourselves and establish spiritual connection to unearth the deeper part of what allowed cancer to manifest in our body. In this book, we will explore the themes of cancer and the common threads of spontaneous remission. Our goal is to explore all of the relational habits, processing habits, beliefs and mindset factors involved in cancer. This will help us understand the following question: what are the big pieces of the puzzle you need to change and address when you have cancer or when you are trying to promote longevity?

By in large, my clients who successfully experience spontaneous remission from cancer have an approach to their diagnosis that is all encompassing. Many times, I ask my clients the question, why do you have cancer? And what needs to change to support your body during this diagnosis? Sometimes my clients just stare at me blankly and say, "I don't know why. My mom had cancer and so did my grandpa. Genes?" Sometimes my clients say something along the lines of this, "Stress. I have so much stress in my life. I have cancer because of stress." Other times, my clients look at me confidently and say the following: "Everything needs to change in my life for me to heal. I am frustrated in my career. I don't have meaningful relationships. I have been semi-abusive to my body because of stress and the lack of time. I am afraid, stressed and lonely most of the time. I know that I need to make some big changes and this diagnosis got my attention. I am ready to change." Is this you? Do you see yourself needing to make big changes to support your body during this diagnosis or to help promote longevity in your life?

Japanese research has discovered that spontaneous remission from cancer occurs within 24-hours of a profound internal transformation.[1] What? A profound, internal transformation. I am going to let you think about that for a few weeks. Just put the book down, think about what I just said every day for a few weeks and then come back to read the rest of this book.

Just kidding. But if I could wrap my head around this phrase: a profound, internal transformation. If I could understand it, implement it and see it manifest, Wow! My life would be vastly different as a result; my understanding of my relationships, my purpose, and myself would be continually changing if I could have the courage to pursue a profound, internal transformation. If you could walk away from this book with one thing, I would hope that you could understand the process that it takes to position yourself to receive a profound, internal transformation.

So, how exactly does someone go through a profound, internal transformation? What does that even mean? Does that mean that someone has surgery and the surgeon removes a few of their organs? That is a profound, internal transformation. No!

A profound, internal transformation is much deeper than your biochemistry. You could call it a paradigm shift. You could call it waking up. You could call it seeing the light. You could call it a revelation. A new relationship with life, a new relationship with you, and new relationships with others can all be keys to a profound, internal transformation. In fact, a profound, internal transformation for you will be vastly different than for your husband, your child, or your best friend. It is unique to YOU; to your maladaptive core beliefs; to your unhealthy emotional processing habits; to the ways that you have protected yourself from being hurt in relationships with others, yourself and even with God/the universe/the divine.

Thus, this book is about renewing your vows. Vows to be good to yourself: that you have value and that you must be cared for as a significant being with untapped potential for bringing good to planet earth. This book is also about renewing your vows to others: to seek others good without harming your own good; to add value to everyone around you; to seek reconciliation whenever possible; to seek understanding instead of assuming motives and becoming offended and hardened towards vulnerable, life-giving relationships. This book is a vow to come alive again when part of you has died, saying no to hope and no to living life by exploring your potential good and releasing your higher purpose to impact those who know you and those who do not know you. It's about leaving a legacy. This book is about connection: finding, renewing and establishing connection with your true identity and relating to yourself, others and the divine in a way that is powerful and opens up the possibility of a profound, internal transformation. Let me show you the path to get there: spontaneous remission is within your reach, just get out your shovel and dig deep with me.

INTRODUCTION

If you don't know anything about me from my other book, *What Is Cancer*, my Cancer Peace University program, my Facebook posts, or You Tube videos, then let me catch you up quickly. I have spent the last 20-years of my life learning the inner depths and wiring of the mind, body, soul and spirit to better serve those with cancer and to help people with incurable diseases experience a profound, internal transformation. I have gone through many profound paradigm shifts myself, have experienced my own healing from an incurable disease, and have seen many experience spontaneous remission from cancer. I am fascinated by and somewhat addicted to the process of understanding the mystery surrounding spontaneous remission from cancer. The more I move away from broccoli as the pinnacle point of the conversation with my cancer clients, and the deeper I seek to impact change in a client's attitude, disposition, mental processing, emotional processing, and connection with self and others, the more I tend to conclude that eating broccoli is probably still a good idea. However, the deeper core transformations tend to ripple through biochemistry in a more profound manner than broccoli ever could. Connection, identity and healing past wounds have become paramount in my work with cancer clients and the purpose of this book is to help you address the deeper core issues in a systematic way. If this doesn't make sense to you right now, I am hoping to make it clearer through the expansion of this book. Follow me to the deeper side of understanding how our biology is wired for spontaneous remission.

How Did I Find My Identity & Purpose?

When I did an internship in Los Angeles, California, I remember trying to join a knitting club. I thought, hey, this might be fun, knit a couple of scarfs and give them to my friends as Christmas gifts, you never know. I tried it for 2 weeks. I found myself dreading the day that knitting club was happening. I stuffed my yarn and knitting sticks in the back of the closet and just wanted to forget all about the whole thing. I learned very quickly that knitting was just not for me. It was not a piece of the puzzle of ME, or what makes me come alive and best express my true self.

When I first went to college at Vanderbilt University, I was pre-med and thought that I was going become a medical doctor. In high school, I had LOVED my chemistry classes, calculus classes and science classes. All of a sudden, in college, I completely lost my passion for chemistry. I found myself hating my chemistry lab and chemistry class. At the same time that I despised chemistry labs, my friends kept on saying to me, "you are the best listener that I have ever met." I kept hearing the same thing over and over again about my gift for listening. It struck a chord in me every time someone acknowledged my ability to listen and show empathy. At some point in the process of discovering my identity, I started to think that I would pursue counseling.

I found out about the 5-year Master's program in Human Development Counseling at Vanderbilt University and signed up for the classes in the second semester of my freshman year. I found my new classes so fascinating that I decided to drop out of pre-med. In the beginning, it felt cloudy and unclear, but as I listened to the message that was coming to me through my natural desires and natural gifting, I started finding a true extension of myself for my career path.

Part of our identity is what we are naturally good at and what we have a natural inclination towards. Another part of our identity seems to be a blueprint for our wiring that we can discover or reject. Some people describe it as our purpose or destiny on Earth. It seems that we can find our purpose bit by bit when we are ready for the next stage. I didn't know that I was going to work with cancer patients when I started my Master's program in counseling. I just knew that I had a gift for listening to people, and I found purpose in helping people process the deep, painful parts of their lives. The purpose of working with cancer patients came many years later. Ironically, it was during moments of my greatest pain and deepest sorrow that I found the additional parts of my identity that gave me the courage to continue pressing forward into discovering and living out my purpose.

"Crisis of Identity"

Many times, it seemed that I would find a piece of myself after a major loss, which I call the "crisis of identity." In these seasons of a crisis of identity, it would feel like part of me was dying and then I would find something that would make me come alive again. For example, when I broke up with my first boyfriend, it felt like part of me died. However, in the midst of the death of part of my soul, I found holistic medicine and became passionate about holistic healing. When my friend Sherry died of cancer, I grieved immensely but birthed my identity in the cancer field and found the greatest calling of my life. When my son, Noble Thomas died, I felt like my arm had been amputated off of my body and that I would never feel whole again, but I received the gift of Cancer Peace University, what my practice is today and saw my work with cancer patients be forever transformed. The collateral beauty that comes from loss and tragedy is an experience that is mysterious and defies human logic, but if we can open our hearts to receive it, we can receive our greatest gifts and puzzle pieces to our identity amidst our darkest days.

You may be walking through your darkest days right now in the midst of a cancer diagnosis. I want to tell you that there is hope. My hope is that in the midst of your crisis of identity that you find who you truly are and what you are meant to do with the one life you have been given.

Section 1: Getting Right with Me

Chapter 1: A Change of Mind: The Journey from Negativity to Positivity is not as far as you Think

Slamming the door of the car behind her, my roommate, Sjhira (pronounced Ji-rah) yelled, "I can't stand being around your negativity any longer. It's so depressing." Shocked, I struggled to understand what was happening and how to respond. I didn't realize that one of my closest friends from college and long-standing roommate felt this way. Me, negative? I'm not negative, I'm in touch with my feelings and I value being authentic. I'm much more concerned about toxic positivity than I am about being slightly negative and realistic while being vulnerable.

"Well, I'm just trying to be honest, is that a crime! I would rather be authentic than be fake and not share my true feelings!" I retorted back and ran up to my room out of confusion and hurt. Through the years of our friendship, I had never gotten into a fight with my friend, Sjhira. Thus, I didn't really know what to do with her revealed feelings towards me. I wasn't a negative person, was I?

I had lived with my friend Sjhira for about 5 years at the time that our first fight happened. It was amazing that we had gone that long without ever fighting about anything besides dishes and cleaning habits. Initially, I found Sjhira to be annoyingly happy and positive. She was THE Pollyanna of Positivity. When we were deciding where to live, for example, she chose the room facing the sunrise so that she could wake up to the sun. I wanted to vomit when she said that out loud. I wanted the room that faced the moon so that I could stay up as late as possible and wake up as late as possible. Thus, her preference worked perfectly for me. If anyone was the exact opposite of me, Sjhira was. In fact, up to that point in my life, I had never had a friend that was so different from me. If Sjhira was THE Pollyanna of Positivity, I was Follow your Feelings Fiona. I was obsessed with noticing and expressing all of my feelings, connecting with the emotions of others, and showing compassion. I did not see any need for positivity. In fact, in feeling all of my feelings and all of the feelings of those around me, I had enough on my plate. And all of those emotions were quite heavy, and leaned me more towards negativity. I did not see how negative I was until I lived with the epitome of positivity.

At the moment the car door slammed, my eyes were opened. I still remember that day. I was shocked into the reality of how I was impacting others. I was trying to be authentic and I didn't want to depress anyone, but I was simply depressed by my own negative thinking.

I became even more aware of my disposition when my friends dubbed me "Melancholy Megan" as an endearing nickname. I didn't want to be "Melancholy Megan", but I also didn't know how to change myself. In fact, it was very difficult to live in my own headspace because I did have a lot of negative thinking. I was very critical of myself. I also felt that my thoughts were very complicated and hard to organize and change.

Despite the fact that our natural dispositions were grating on one another at times, Sjhira and I were and still are the best of friends. We have been there for each other at the highest moments and the lowest moments of life, and living together was actually a life-changing experience for both of us.

Near the end of living together for almost 5 years, people began to comment that Sjhira and I looked alike. Physically, there were not a lot of similarities between Sjhira and I. In fact, Sjhira was black and I was white. I had blue/green eyes and Sjhira had brown eyes. I had straight hair and Sjhira had naturally curly hair. However, living together for 5 years, we started to have similar mannerisms, hand gestures, jokes and expressions. And strangely enough, I felt slightly more positive.

It wasn't until we moved away from each other for over 6 months that we both noticed striking differences in our thinking and way of relating with ourselves and others. Sjhira called me, laughing while she said, "I feel different. I think that your compassion rubbed off on me! Is that possible?"

I laughed as well and said, "you know what? I actually think that I am more positive than I have ever been in my life. Thank you for slamming the door on me that day and telling me how negative I was. I think it really did something. Shock therapy in its best form!"

This is an example of what it means when people say, "the best lessons in life are caught and not taught." I truly caught something so valuable from Sjhira. I found out that it is possible to feel all of your feelings and to be positive at the same time. I also began a lifelong process of rewiring my brain towards positivity. It was such a relief to not be destined to a life of being "Melancholy Megan."

Back to my story of Sjhira slamming the car door on me. You may have heard my story about sleeping towards the moon and feeling annoyed around uber positive people and thought, that is me, too! Or you may have heard my story and thought; I can't even believe that this is possible, that you can change so dramatically! It takes commitment, honest introspection and shifting your paradigm of beliefs over and over again, but you can do this! Your brain is wired to be rewired over and over again, until it is healthy, positive and strong! Let's explore the scientific term neuroplasticity, which is what I experienced in living with Sjhira.

Our thinking and disposition has real consequences on our health. In fact, a study published in *The Journal of National Cancer Institute* in 1998 found that women who experienced long-term depression were 90% more likely to develop cancer than peers who were more positive.[1] Do I have Sjhira to thank for a boost towards more positive health outcomes in my life? Quite possibly.

Prior to experiencing my brain change, I didn't think that I had much choice in my thinking and negative disposition. In fact, I felt like a helpless victim of negative thinking. I felt like my brain had been hijacked because of my natural gift of empathy. I simply thought, with every gift, there is a drawback. My drawback was negative thinking from the weight of emotional intelligence and connection. However, this was simply not true. I didn't realize that I actually had a choice in my thoughts and that I could stand outside of my thoughts as an observer and decide to make changes in my thinking.

Dr. Kristin Neff, a researcher and professor at The University of Texas at Austin studies self-compassion and defines self-compassion as developing the following three traits: 1. Self-kindness: Be warm and understanding towards yourself when you fail, feel inadequate or when you suffer. 2. Common Humanity: Instead of feeling alone in your suffering, feelings of inadequacy and suffering is a common thread through humanity and the message is that you are not alone. 3. Mindfulness: Don't suppress or exaggerate emotions. Make sure to identify and express thoughts and emotions in a balanced way by learning to not ignore pain, but also to not over-identify with thoughts and feelings. If you over-identify with your thoughts and feelings, you can be over-swept with negativity.[2] This was exactly my problem. I had begun to over-identify with my thoughts and feelings and this exaggeration created patterns of negative thinking with a general disposition towards negativity. I had to swing the other direction and learn to find a balance, shifting my brain towards a healthy state of optimism.

In the 1980s, the focus surrounding the brain was compensation. If neurologists, psychiatrists and health practitioners could alter the brain chemistry to allow for changes, we may see some benefits and compensation for the lack of optimal brain function. Full restoration of brain function was not believed to be possible at that time. However, neuroplasticity has become the norm of understanding the brain in research and in practical application. In fact, therapies geared towards total brain restoration as opposed to brain compensation have come on the forefront of cutting edge treatments for the brain.

The research and results of these types of treatment point towards a powerful concept in our brains: our brains are plastic and can be rewired towards optimal function. Neuroplasticity means that our brains are malleable and adaptable, even changing moment by moment of every day. Neurogenesis means that every morning when you wake up, new baby nerve cells have been born while you were sleeping and you have an opportunity to rebuild healthy thoughts while tearing down toxic thoughts.[3]

How do our thoughts impact our biology and correlate with a cancer diagnosis? Our thought patterns literally impact the expression of DNA. Eric Kandel, a

Nobel-Prize winning neuro-psychiatrist found that thoughts and imaginations get under the skin of our DNA and can turn genes on and off changing the structure of neurons in the brain.[4] Epigenetics is a fairly new field of study that examines signals that trigger the silencing and expression of our DNA.[5] Epigenetics means "upon the genes." Signal molecules coming from emotions, beliefs, thought patterns and nutrition act to unzip DNA and can have either a positive impact on our biology or a negative one.[6]

75-98% of mental, physical and behavioral illness comes from one's thought life, whereas only 2-25% of mental, physical and behavioral illness comes from the environment and genes.[7] Further, a study performed at HeartMath found that thinking and feeling anger, fear, and frustration caused DNA to change shape accordingly, the DNA became tight and much shorter while turning off some DNA. However, this was reversed when the person began to generate feelings of love, joy, appreciation and gratitude.[8]

In this first section, we are seeking to understand how to shift our relationship with ourselves. We are laying the foundation in understanding how our brains are wired to change based upon input, learning, meditation, and standing outside of ourselves to challenge our thought processes. Our brains are not fixed and static; rather, the study of neuroplasticity has demonstrated that our brains are wired to adapt based upon learning and creating new brain connections and networks. In fact, neuroplasticity has shown that the brain can be rewired towards a positive disposition even in the most negative brain space (like mine when I lived with Sjhira). In order to have a profound, internal transformation, you may need to "get right with yourself" by starting to examine your thinking and change your thoughts towards yourself.

We have the unique ability to stand outside of ourselves, observe our thoughts about others and ourselves and decide to change our thinking. In addition, dealing with childhood wounds, releasing the past, forgiving and releasing regrets will be other steps that we will take in the process of building a new relationship with yourself throughout this book.

In order to pursue a right relationship with yourself, the following qualities need to be developed:

1. Honesty and integrity with yourself and others. If you cannot be honest with yourself and those you trust, you will struggle to succeed. Deceiving and lying to yourself and trying to protect yourself from the truth (the truth hurts sometimes!), will stifle this process. If you want an easy, quick fix, without having to suffer or learn something negative about yourself, then you can continue to lie to yourself and decide to not change.

I could have easily ignored Sjhira's frustrations on the day that she slammed the door and called me out on my negativity. I could have stubbornly refused to look at the feedback I was receiving. Most of the time, the very thing that needs to change is out of our vantage point, in the blind spot of our lives and in order to see the place of our greatest need to change, we need to receive some honest feedback from close friends and family members. First of all, we need to allow people close enough to give appropriate feedback to trigger changes in our understanding. Many of us isolate and create roadblocks to these types of relationships.

Secondly, we need to be open to receive that feedback in the right moments in a way that allows us to change. The first question is: do you have people in your life to give you feedback in an honest way? Have you allowed people close enough? Why or why not? If you don't have close relationships or you have been hurt in the past and have closed yourself off to this type of relationship, you may need to decide to open up again and allow people close enough.

2. A willingness to change and humility to acknowledge your need to change. Some people have a stubborn streak and it will take the worst pain ever to address a physical or emotional ailment. I definitely have a stubborn streak as well as a history of repeating the same behaviors over and over again, expecting different results. The definition of insanity is: doing the same thing over and over again, expecting different results. Why do we as humans do this? We know from experience that the last time we ate the entire tub of ice cream, we felt sick and wanted to vomit, so why did we just do it again? If you want to get out of behavioral cycles of insanity, you will need a strong dose of humility and a willingness to change.

3. A hunger to live a free and passionate life. Those who want to live a unique life must get to know themselves, allow themselves to change, heal and recover from the past to step into a promising future.

4. An intensity and willingness to do what it takes and to commit to the ups and downs of the process. Developing a healthy relationship with yourself does not happen overnight and it takes commitment, perseverance and an intensity that not all people have. Let's get started now that we have some basic understanding of neuroplasticity and have thought through some deeper questions about ourselves. Get ready to dig deep and rewire your brain towards health, love, and optimism.

There are so many self-help books out there and many of them are excellent; however, not all of them provide the opportunity to experience a profound, internal transformation. Working on your relationship with yourself and others, as well as dealing with past trauma and deepening spiritual connection throughout this book will pave the way towards that profound, internal shift that you are seeking. However, much of the work will be in how you apply the new knowledge that this book is offering to you. We suggest that you work on applying the knowledge by purchasing and doing the exercises in Braving The Storm Companion Workbook: In Pursuit Of A Profound, Internal Transformation. At this point, you can open your companion workbook and begin to go through the exercises for Section 1: Getting Right with Me, Chapter 1: A Change Of Mind.

Section 1: Getting Right with Me

Chapter 2: Releasing Regret & Shame: I Am Not My Worst Mistake

Throwing myself on my bed, I sobbed tears of regret, shame and remorse. I couldn't believe that I let things get so out of control. What is wrong with me?

I heard the door of my room open and my heart nearly jumped out of my chest. I turned my head to the door and tried to brush my tangled hair out of my eyes, but there was no use. I was a mess. I saw my dad at the door and just the look in his face was enough to completely break my heart. Complete and utter disappointment. He didn't need to say anything, I just knew. "Megan, I am so disappointed in you. If only you would have asked me, I would have bought you the make-up. I don't understand. We didn't raise you like this. I just don't know how I can trust you after this," my dad uttered the worst words I could have heard from him as a teenager. As quickly as he opened the door to share these piercing daggers, he slid out of the door and I was left to my shame and regret.

Sobbing, I replayed the last few months in my head to try to understand how I had arrived at this point. I remembered my friend saying to me a few weeks ago, "I'm done with shoplifting, I think it's getting out of control and we need to stop." Part of me agreed with her, however, the other part of me didn't want to let it go. I finally felt socially accepted. Thinking about last year, I could still wince in pain of rejection when I remembered the days that I ran to the bathroom stall to eat lunch in order to avoid rejection when trying to choose a table of peers to join for lunch. Being in 8th grade had been brutal, especially during lunch. There was the cool table, with all the beautiful and popular kids where I definitely knew I didn't belong. And there was the funny and cool table with the athletic and personable types. Sometimes there was a spot for me and sometimes there wasn't. And some days, I could just not bear the stress of finding a table to belong to and to feel welcome. So, I would sit in the bathroom stall by myself and feel so much shame and rejection. What was wrong with me and why was it so hard to be accepted?

The summer before 9th grade, I grew taller, lost some weight and got my braces off. In general, I blossomed in some socially acceptable ways. I also got my license earlier than others at the beginning of 10th grade and got my own car. Getting into the right social cliché became easier all of a sudden. The undercurrent of rejection, shame and fear didn't lift so easily though and when my friends thought it was cool to shoplift and slightly pressured me to follow suit, I wasn't going to be the odd person out. I played my part.

A couple of weeks after one of my friends ended her shoplifting habit, another friend and I went to Target before going to see the newly released movie, The Titanic. While in Target, my friend and I stole some make-up and a watch. Laughing and running from the store, we were not at all expecting to be caught. This scene had played over a dozen of times at different stores at the local mall and nothing had happened, until now. A man followed closely behind us and asked us a seemingly innocent question, "what time is it?" We turned to respond and quickly realized that this wasn't a casual interaction. The man turned out to be the security guard for Target and we were caught red-handed.

After this event occurred, I did some deep soul searching. I realized a few things:

1. I wasn't as "good" of a person as I thought I was. I had thought I was a good person because I had straight A's in school, I made sure to sign up for community service, I had built up a fairly good resume, I had some close friends and I was fairly athletic, playing several different types of sports. All of the reasons that I thought I was a good person were not adding up when I was caught shop-lifting and broke trust with my parents. I needed to figure out what it really meant to be a "good person."

2. I didn't want to disappoint my dad ever again and I needed to rebuild trust.

3. I didn't want to live for the attention and affirmation of my peers, especially when it led to destructive behaviors.

There were many consequences to being caught shoplifting at Target including:

1. Community Service
2. Attending classes about stealing with my mother, which was terribly mortifying as I was in a class with hardened criminals and people who had a history of stealing cars, robbing banks and more.
3. Being banned from the local Target store for the rest of my life.

I chose to do community service at the Lutheran church next to my high school. I met the high school minister and his wife and they invited me to become a church counselor at the high school camp that happened every summer. Me, a church camp counselor? I don't think you know whom you are asking. I felt completely unworthy to play this role. I was far away from saint status and had just been caught performing a criminal act. I was uncertain and felt completely unqualified.

The weight of the external consequences was not as heavy as the daily mental and emotional toil within my soul. I was wrestling deeply with some things that I didn't fully understand at the time and that would take me many years to uncover the depths of my shame and sense of unworthiness.

Layer by layer, I began to unwrap that question in my soul, what is wrong with me? In addition, this question led me to ask another question, what is right with me? And how do we define morality? Are we inherently good, inherently bad or a mixture of both? And who decides this? I didn't realize at the time that I was in the middle of a basic worldview conflict and I would need to go through a paradigm shift in my beliefs to answer the questions that loomed deep in my soul.

That summer, when I served as a camp counselor, I was struck so deeply by one of the sermons that I cried and cried until my soul felt cleansed. I longed for a new beginning. That camp trip marked a fresh start that continued as I decided to go out of state for college the year after my senior year.

I Am Not My Worst Mistake

This was the beginning of a profound new journey that led me deeper into a healthy relationship with others and myself as well as into a deep spiritual connection. As Carl Jung stated: *"I am not what has happened to me (or what I have done). I am what I choose to become."* From the moment that I was caught shoplifting until now, I chose a path of change and healing. Now I can tell this story with no shame as it quite literally feels like another lifetime in which I did not exist.

Everyone experiences shame, regret and the feeling of just not being enough. We have seasons and moments where we feel that we are wrong, are bad and are inherently a mess. How do we move past the shame that we feel and the regrets that we carry? If we carry shame and hide from others, and ourselves we have a disconnected part of our life that causes us to lose integrity in our identity. If we can find empathy in the midst of our shame, by finding that we are not alone, that we are not judged and that we can find connection at our lowest points, then we find freedom from shame.

I was able to find freedom from shame by connecting with the high school ministers at the Lutheran church. Shame and condemnation thrive in secrets and in hiding. James Pennebaker and a team of psychologists at The University of Texas studied what happened when survivors of rape and incest kept their experiences a secret. The research team found that withholding their experience from others through secrecy was actually more damaging than the event itself.[1] On the other hand, when people shared their trauma with others, their physical health improved, their doctor's visits decreased and they showed a decrease in stress hormones. [2]

Many people find it hard to connect in a vulnerable way with loved ones and express deep pain and feelings of inadequacy. We have learned to hide our pain, suppress our emotions and wear a mask that says, "I'm fine, don't ask me how I am really doing." How many of us have endured the painful times of adolescence and learned to hide our true selves out of fear of being rejected or shamed?

Brene Brown, a vulnerability and shame expert, has researched the many different ways we try to hide our shame and disconnect from people to protect ourselves. She found that people learn to protect themselves from emotional pain in three different ways:[3]

1. Foreboding Joy: to avoid perpetually being disappointed, many people don't fully embrace moments of joy, but rehearse tragedy as a way to prepare themselves for the "other shoe to drop."

2. **Perfectionism:** this is an attempt to earn approval based upon the belief that if we do things perfectly, we can minimize pain, shame, judgment and mistakes.

3. **Numbing:** we numb pain and trauma by being too busy to think or feel, using drugs, food, alcohol, caffeine and substances to numb pain.

The problem with these three strategies is that we don't deal with our root feelings of shame, condemnation, inadequacy or lack of worthiness. We simply avoid feeling deep emotions by avoiding authentic connection and expression of our true feelings.

Brene Brown discovered several strategies to help move from a place of hiding or protecting ourselves to developing authentic vulnerability. *Instead of rehearsing the worst-case scenario, developing a gratitude practice helps to focus our brains around what we have and what brings us joy on a daily basis.* Some people find it helpful to keep a gratitude journal to help enhance their joy and gratefulness in small moments surrounding daily life. To be effective in building a grateful attitude, inviting joy and rejecting the tendency to prepare for the worst, write down 3 things that you are grateful for every morning or evening. Make sure that you write down very specific and unique gratitude's rather than general ones like, 1. I am alive. 2. I woke up. 3. I have food and a house.

It is most helpful to focus on very specific and unique gratitude's like the following: 1. I am grateful for the moment in the day when I connected with my son and we sang his favorite song together and were laughing at the dance moves that we were making during the song. 2. I am grateful that my husband made my favorite meal for dinner, fish tacos. 3. I am grateful that my mom comes to help with my son once a week so that I can work on my business. Every day, focus on newly discovered gratitude's to build your gratitude practice.

To deal with perfectionism, we need to first realize the drawbacks of perfectionistic tendencies. Research shows that perfectionism hampers achievement and leads to life paralysis, fear of failing, depression, anxiety and addictive behaviors. When did you believe the lie that "you are what you accomplish and how well you accomplish it?" Perfectionism is more about the perception of other people than it is about our accomplishments. Realistically, we cannot control another person's perception of us. **In order to recover from perfectionism, we need to start creating.** I know that I am in a positive life flow when I am not afraid to try new things or to be creative. I remember when I came home from living in Cape Town, South Africa in 2010. I started to go Lindy Hop dancing as a new social and athletic outlet. In the beginning stages, I was really, really bad at it. But, I had so much fun, and I was laughing through all of my mistakes and inadequacies during the dance. I felt free from perfectionism when I started to Lindy Hop as I improvised and created with my body and my dance partner. **Over time, I slowly improved my skills, but I still never dance perfectly. However, I am creating when I dance and when I am creating something, I feel a sense of joy and freedom.**

In order to deal with the tendency to numb pain from a sense of inadequacy, we can learn to set up the appropriate boundaries so that we are taking on only the amount of responsibility that we can handle. When we become too busy to think, we are driven to strive and to numb out the shame and anxiety by fulfilling the requirements that are asked of us without boundaries. However, when we set up boundaries, we respect our own limitations and are better able to manage the tasks and responsibilities that are within our capability. **We draw a line around our value and let the world know that I will do my best to fulfill**

my responsibility, but I will not sacrifice the well being of my family and myself in order to perform my way into recognition.

In his book, Writing to Heal, Pennebaker states the following: "Since the mid-1980s an increasing number of studies have focused on the value of expressive writing as a way to bring about healing. The evidence is mounting that the act of writing about traumatic experiences for as little as 15-20 minutes a day for 3-4 days can produce measurable changes in physical and mental health. Emotional writing can also affect people's sleep habits, work efficiency, and how they connect with others."[4]

I will share more on my personal journey to finding deep personal, relational and spiritual connection as this book unfolds. For now, in line with Pennebaker's research, let's do a writing exercise in your companion workbook. As important as it is to have the knowledge to understand how to change and what leads to a profound, internal transformation, we need to take some practical steps. Use this book not only as a guide, a tool, and a source of knowledge, but also as an exercise and an opportunity to "get right with yourself."

Section 1: Getting Right with Me

Chapter 3: Freeing Your Mind from Imprints of Trauma

Zigzagging through the bustling movement of college students running late to class, I briefly looked up in the distance and my heart skipped a beat as Joe, my new "friend" was heading straight towards me with a warm smile on his face.

Feeling light-headed and slightly nauseous, I stopped mid-step and gave a faint, "Hey, what's up?" secretly hoping that he wasn't rushing off to class and had some time to chat.

I wasn't about to hurry off to my lunch meeting with my friend, Sara. She could wait, it wasn't every day that I found myself running into Joe, the sweet, kind and magnetic friend that I just couldn't stop thinking about lately. "Hey, Megan, what are you up to?" Joe asked, casually.

"Not much just finished class." I feigned a relaxed, I'm not late to a lunch meeting right now, low-key stance.

An hour later, tears brimming in my eyes, I shared with Joe some of my deepest fears regarding my recent diagnosis of Polycystic Ovary Syndrome (PCOS). He was so easy to talk to. Without a word, I felt his tender, compassionate heart making room for some of the more vulnerable feelings that I was carrying. I had some massive concerns regarding my ability to have children in the future with my recent diagnosis of PCOS and I hadn't felt the freedom to talk about it with people in my life, until I met Joe. He was the type of person that was so trustworthy, I felt heard and known by him even though we had only met a few months prior.

We had many things in common, and our friendship, or whatever it was, felt completely natural and meant to be. The strange thing that I noticed around this time was that I naturally opened up to my guy friends, but my female friends I kept at a distance. I just couldn't unwrap the layers of my emotions with my female friends in the way that I could with Joe and other guy friends of mine.

It became a nagging concern, over time, as I found myself spending more and more time with my guy friends and less and less time with women. I couldn't pinpoint why, but I felt uneasy and devoid of emotion around women, whereas I found myself sharing my deepest pain with male friends. When my female friends opened up about emotions or asked me about my emotions, I felt like a brick wall. I began to ask myself the questions: "Why do I do this? Why can I open up to my friends that are guys, but I can't open up to women?"

The answer came like a miraculous revelation that left me shocked and in a tailspin of emotions. At that time, I was journaling, discovering my emotions and developing my emotional intelligence. One day, when I was journaling and listening to Enya, my meditative music of choice at the time, I saw a memory play before me that was strangely familiar. I saw myself in 2nd grade. I hadn't recalled this memory so when the images played before me, it felt like I was watching a movie about myself that was strangely familiar and distant at the same time.

Before I share the memory, I will say that I had an idyllic, wonderful childhood. I had everything that I needed and my parents were wonderful. I share this memory to show that even in the best of childhoods, there are situations that occur that skew our perception of reality based upon how we interpret what happens to us. In the memory, I saw myself struggling with my body image and trying to open up to my mom about how I was feeling. One way that we would bond would be to go shopping and buy new clothes before the school year. I looked forward to that time every year as we would spend the whole day shopping together and would eat lunch at the mall. It was always a joyful event. However, this particular year, the clothes were not fitting right and I felt fat. Being a gymnast and a dancer, I compared myself to all of my friends who were super skinny. I started crying, feeling deeply afraid of rejection and pain surrounding my body image.

As I saw my little self-crying and vulnerable, saying something to the effect of, "the clothes aren't fitting me right." My mother's practical advice to me, at that time, felt like a harsh critique, "I think you need to stop eating so much ice cream." My little face fell in shame and I sucked up every emotion inside of myself and made a decision in that moment: I decided that I would not cry in front of women ever again. From that day forward, I never cried in front of a female again.

My mother was merely giving me a solution to my problem, as well as trying to instill a principle that if I wanted things to change, I would have to put in some effort. A very basic and practical step; however, my young heart couldn't process those words as constructive because deep down, I just wanted a hug. I wanted my feelings to be validated. I longed to feel understood, loved, and heard. Ultimately, I wanted connection to cover the shame that I felt about my body.

As soon as I realized the decision that I had made on that fateful day, I saw flashes of memories where I would run from women in tears to hide my emotions and sadness from them. I saw myself at figure skating competitions running from my mom and skating coach to the bathroom to cry when I was disappointed in my performance. I saw myself in 2nd grade, running from my 2nd grade teacher to cry in the bathroom. I saw myself in high school running up the stairs to my room, throwing myself on my bed sobbing after being rejected by a classmate whom I asked to Homecoming, hiding my tears from my mom. I even remember my mom knocking on my door in frustration saying, "Why won't you let me in?" At the time, I didn't know why I wouldn't cry in front of my mom or any other female.

All of a sudden, it all made sense. In this memory, I believed that I could not trust females with my deep emotions, and as a result I decided to stop crying in front of women. I made an inner vow or inner decision to protect myself from being hurt again. It worked until I was in college and realized that my relationships with women were suffering as a result of this decision. I wanted to be vulnerable with women again and I was ready to take the plunge.

This was the answer to my pattern of relating to females differently than males, and now that I knew, I could do something about it! When we have vivid memories that come into our conscious awareness, we can redesign them and actually shift any behavioral patterns that we have developed as a result of our "maladaptive core beliefs."

From the womb to age 7, you develop your worldview or your belief system, which consists of the beliefs you carry that allow you to interpret the world around you. Your belief system is stored in your subconscious mind and can be found imprinted in your memories. To create your belief system, you make conclusions based upon life experiences and these conclusions become your core beliefs. Not every conclusion is good or even based upon reality, thus, some of our beliefs become maladaptive.

For example, if you experience rejection as a child, you can process the rejection in a healthy way and conclude something positive or you can develop a maladaptive core belief based upon the experience of rejection. Children who have parents who can help them process rejection or other emotions can help keep fleeting moments from defining them in a negative way. However, if you experience rejection and are unable to process it or find help from an adult in your life, you may end up coming to the conclusion that you are rejected. This can become a maladaptive core belief that will guide your worldview and make you actually expect rejection in life. Your thought patterns and emotions in present day reality would then mirror your belief that you are rejected and you will experience rejection over and over again, until you address and shift your belief system away from this maladaptive core belief.

Core beliefs in the subconscious mind arising from childhood trauma can be altered and rewritten in order to shift the epigenetic factors of disease. These factors include beliefs, thought patterns and emotions of trauma, abuse and neglect. The Default Mode Network is the paradigm or worldview that was developed in our subconscious mind throughout our childhood.

When I became aware of this memory from childhood, I forgave my mother in the memory and made a new decision to open up to females again. Immediately, everything changed. I found myself blubbering in front of my friends who were females, and I felt free! It was an amazing experience because it was such a dramatic shift in my beliefs and my behavior all at once.

Let's explore more about the role of childhood trauma and illness. Childhood trauma can be strongly linked to present day illness. The majority of my clients with cancer have unresolved childhood trauma or trauma that occurred several months to a few years prior to their cancer diagnosis. In fact, a study performed by Fecitti and Anda found 10 types of adverse childhood experiences (ACEs) that were correlated with present day illness. This longitudinal study on ACEs had 17,000 participants over 2 years, each taking physical exams with interviews about their childhood experiences.[1]

Abuse, neglect, losing a parent, witnessing domestic violence, living with someone with a mental illness, drug dependency, and constant low-level stress of emotional neglect were all major predictors for obesity, cancer and heart disease.

Only half of ACE-related illnesses correlate to disease-causing behaviors used to cope after experiencing trauma or chronic stress from childhood. The other half of ACE-related illness correlates to the reality that stress and trauma in childhood can rewrite your DNA, recoding your body to be more susceptible to disease.

I will give you an example from a client of mine. I worked with a client who was diagnosed with col-rectal cancer. She had many aspects of healing that we were working on together. One day, it came to light that she had nearly drowned when she was only 3 years old! I also found out that on a regular basis, she would imagine herself dying. For example, if she were to drive over a bridge, she would imagine her car crashing off the side of the bridge and her drowning in the lake beneath. In addition, when she would drive home from work and no one was home, sometimes she would imagine a person inside her house with a gun, ready to shoot her. We realized that she had an imprint of death upon her because of the experience of nearly drowning when she was only 3 years old. We redesigned her memory of almost drowning and she was able to move forward without the strong imaginations of death around every corner.

Thus, the clues to our core beliefs are daily thought patterns, emotional patterns, and relational patterns. Once a pattern comes to your awareness, asking a question like, "What is connected to this pattern in my life," can lead you to an answer in the form of a memory from your subconscious mind.

You can start tracing patterns internally or externally. If you start internally, journaling is an important tool to track and recognize thought patterns and emotional patterns. It is easiest to trace and follow a dominant emotion to a memory that carries a maladaptive core belief. Sometimes, to find the dominant emotion, we need to start by free-association journaling. This means that you journal all of your thoughts 15-20 minutes a day without editing, judging or analyzing. Simply write down your thoughts as they come to you.

Allow yourself to relax and follow your thoughts until you experience the emotion connected to your thought patterns. Once you have the dominant emotion, allow your mind to wander and write down what associations you find. You may discover a memory that you haven't thought about for a while or access a memory in your subconscious mind that you have not consciously held since it occurred. Now you are ready to redesign your memory. Explore how you felt in the memory at every point and try to discern what you concluded in the memory and what belief you held after the experience. Are there people you need to forgive? Do you need to forgive yourself? Did you make any inner decisions that changed your personality and how you relate to others? Forgiveness within a memory is a powerful strategy to dissipate intense emotions and to change the imprint of the memory. Making new decisions in the memory is also a powerful exercise to shift relating and emotional processing habits.

If you want to explore the external route at the same time or instead of the internal route, start noticing relational patterns in your life. How do you relate to your friends, family, men and women? Do you relate differently depending on whom you are relating to? Why? Is there any memory associated with the way that you relate with men, women, family or friends?

The myth with self-help is that if we can correct our habits or bad behaviors, we can get different results. I have found this impossibly untrue in my life.

Behavioral modification most easily flows out of a profound, internal transformation, shifting a maladaptive core belief, forgiving and redesigning memories.

It is important to understand how our brain works and to approach healing from a place of understanding. Your subconscious mind contains many keys to your healing. In fact, your subconscious mind knows what is necessary for you to experience spontaneous remission from cancer or any other disease that you have. Another term for the subconscious mind is the Default Mode Network (DMN).[2] Disrupting the DMN plays a large role in spontaneous healing. Many people leave their subconscious beliefs about themselves unexamined and thus, beliefs created during their formative years remain fixed. However, we all have the opportunity to challenge any maladaptive core beliefs from childhood by engaging the DMN.

The DMN is a collection of connected areas in the brain that can be activated when we engage in a certain way of thinking. Daydreaming, deep thinking about yourself and others, remembering things that happened in the past, and imagining what might happen in the future all work together to engage the DMN. Introspection and awareness of your emotions also allow the activation of the DMN. Your DMN carries the blueprint of you and how you uniquely operate in the world. Our perception of ourselves can be skewed because of maladaptive core beliefs, thus twisting our identity into a direction that is not positive or healthy. Everyone has some maladaptive beliefs that may or may not be challenged during their lifetime. DMN works best when we spend time integrating past, present and future perceptions of self and spend the appropriate time in deep, introspective thinking. Ultimately, your DMN carries a story that links your past with the present and future in a cohesive and dynamic way that allows the opportunity to challenge negative core beliefs from our past.[3]

If we automatically see ourselves as damaged, wrong, broken, disempowered and unworthy, then we will choose behaviors that reflect that belief system. In order to challenge the DMN and go through a paradigm shift, we need to engage in deep thinking, meditation, journaling, emotional intelligence growth, and memory redesigning. When we engage the activity of the DMN through deep introspection, gamma wave activity increases which correlates with attention, memory building, and learning. In addition, in a gamma wave state, areas of the brain linked to happiness and peace activate.[4]

When someone engages in a deep state of introspection, brain imaging experiments have shown background activity in the brain surrounding recollections, ruminations, imaginations, self-perceptions, and focusing on specific memories.[5] This activity helps to create flexibility, creativity and the ability to plan for the future in the brain.[6] Further, when we engage our DMN, we can gain access to memories in the subconscious mind that we may not have had conscious recollection of for years! These are the beginning stages of accessing memories that hold maladaptive core beliefs, and are keys to experiencing a profound, internal transformation. We cannot gain access to these memories without engaging our DMN through deep thinking, meditation, journaling and being open to discovering what the subconscious mind holds as truth.

The Default Mode Network and healing through a profound, internal transformation is best understood through an example of a client of mine who I will name Josh. Josh came to me with a diagnosis of adrenocortical cancer or adrenal cancer. A rare form of cancer, Josh wanted to do all that he could to avoid the 80% chance the doctor gave him of the tumor returning in a few years. My client, Josh, began to watch the videos in CPU on the Default Mode Network and emotional roots to cancer.

All of a sudden, he stopped the video and knew exactly why he had cancer. He accessed a memory from his childhood that he had not thought about for years. When he was in 3rd grade, he had a crush on a girl in his class. To impress her, he decided to go up to her and tell her a joke. He walked up to Shanna and said, "Hey Shanna, what do you get when you come across a lama and a snake? A dead lama." In his head, the joke was hilarious. However, Shanna looked at him, sneered, and walked away. Josh was devastated. He still remembers going home and ruminating about this rejection for days. It was a defining moment, in a negative way, in his life. Josh felt like a loser, and became more introverted and less spontaneous. He just didn't think that people liked him and he started to people please to gain the approval of others. This skewed his personality. Now, as an adult, he could see how he compromised his own identity.

It was best illuminated to him in his marriage. Everything about his marriage was set up to help his wife feel good about their life together. He literally did not share his deepest desires and opinions about things. At that moment, it was all crystal clear for Josh. He had a lot of changing to do. We redesigned the memory; he made new choices in the memory, forgave himself and Shanna, and in the end, Josh felt like the memory lost its negative hold on his life. From there, Josh had a series of serious conversations with his wife to address the underlying things that he was actually not happy about in their lives. He committed to being authentic and overcoming his fear of losing the approval of others. From that point on, Josh's whole life and perception of himself changed. **This is a profound, internal transformation that starts and ends with engaging the DMN in the brain!**

Research shows that when we don't engage our DMN, we may experience negative self-esteem, depression, worry, anxiety, health issues, short-term memory issues and develop a tendency to focus on the problem instead of the solution.[7] The Task Positive Network (TPN) balances out our Default Mode Network. The TPN is engaged during active thinking required for making decisions.[8] The DMN and TPN are meant to be in balance and when one network is too active with the other becoming more dormant, our brain can suffer the effects of toxic, negative thinking. When we have increased activity of the DMN without shifting into TPN and acting upon our deep thinking, we can develop maladaptive, depressive ruminations and a decreased ability to solve problems, leaving us confused, negative, and depressed. In fact, brain research has discovered that action completes the cycle of building up and breaking down thoughts.[9] Thus, we can either over-engage the DMN, lacking proactivity and engagement after deep thinking or we can lack deep introspection and overly rely upon the TPN. Either of which leads to imbalances mentally that affect our emotional and physical health.

Prior to college, I overly engaged my TPN and was too busy to develop my DMN. I was not a very deep thinker at that time. However, when I started to have panic attacks, my emotional life got my attention and mirrored to me that something was off balance. Once I learned how to engage my DMN, I became depressed because I was overly introspective with little or no proactive step at the end of my deep thinking. Now, I have learned how to balance the two networks in a positive manner.

To set the stage for effective engagement with neuroplasticity, it helps to open the mind by getting out of our daily routine, and learning something new and in turn, creating new neural pathways for the brain. When I began the process of connecting with my subconscious mind, it was very helpful for me to move to Nashville, to start college, and to be in a new environment with new patterns to challenge my DMN.

This was the first time in my life that I learned to slow down and engage in deeply introspective habits like journaling, meditating, and processing all of my thoughts and feelings on a daily basis. In the beginning, it was a messy and confusing process, but over time, it became natural and now something that I engage in all the time without thinking.

People who are diagnosed with cancer often times benefit from making major life changes in areas of their lives in which they carry a lot of frustration in order to assist in their healing process. Many times, my clients will quit their jobs and start a new career path. Or they may move to a new location, travel or learn something new that they have always wanted to learn. They make changes that will not only cause them to find more meaning, but also to lessen daily frustration and to break them free of their DMN that may need a major reset.

If you are new at engaging your DMN in a purposeful manner or if you already journal, meditate and self-reflect, then set aside the time necessary to engage with the exercises in the companion workbook to set the stage for a profound, internal transformation.

Section 1: Getting Right with Me

Chapter 4: Embracing Your Eccentricity

"Hola, Como estas? Me llamo Megan. Como te llamas?" I spoke each word with extra emphasis as I tried my hardest to listen and decipher a response from my new friends, "something... something Pololo." I struggled to capture the essence of this friendly introduction. Frustrated and humiliated, I couldn't believe that I had been studying Spanish for 7 years and I still couldn't manage a proper introduction in Chilean Spanish. Granted, I just arrived last week to Santiago, Chile, but 7 years? You would think that I would be fluent by now.

"Hola, Pololo, mucho gusto?" I spoke timidly, uncertain that I knew what I had heard. Laughing in delight and slight embarrassment for me, I could tell that I picked up the wrong name. I thought that he said his name was Pololo, but from their reaction, clearly, I was wrong. I later learned that Pololo in Chilean Spanish meant boyfriend. So, I had essentially said, "hello, boyfriend, nice to meet you." So embarrassing. This would be the first of many humiliating moments as I attempted to become fluent in Spanish, which was one of my majors at Vanderbilt University. I had been waiting all of 7 years for this moment to study abroad and become fully immersed in Spanish. I still remember when my first Spanish instructor had spoken about studying abroad when I was in 8th grade and here I was, 7 years later.

I love the Spanish language and I love the culture. I went out salsa dancing with my friends and found every opportunity that I could to spend time with native Chileans in order to practice my language skills and experience the culture. Despite the struggle to learn the language, the headaches that I experienced every night before going to bed, and the humiliation of talking like a 2-year-old, I felt more alive than I had in months. There was something about the experience of traveling, living in another culture and interacting with native Chileans that made my soul feel alive and free. It was like catching a breath of air after suffocating or nearly drowning. I felt the most like me than I had for a long time. I emphasized every memory in my brain to ensure that I would always remember what it was like to find myself again.

I couldn't quite put my finger on it, but there was something unique about this trip for me that seemed different than others in my group. Most of the students in my study abroad group spent time together, going to dinner, traveling on the weekends and socializing, but that wasn't what I wanted out of my experience. I was the most joyous surrounded by natives, trying to decipher their intriguing words and their fascinating way of being that was simply different from my own. It was exhilarating beyond anything I had experienced up until that point in my life.

The process of discovering your unique language, your unique fingerprint or your unique identity is challenging. It's like following clues to a buried treasure, but you haven't seen the map. You feel it out, try things, hate it and stop it, try something new, love it, keep it, then do it over and over again because it is a piece of YOU. In the last 39 years of my life, I have tried a lot of things, and I have learned to notice when something clicks into place or when it just feels awkward or too hard to embrace.

When I did an internship in Los Angeles, California, I remember trying to join a knitting club. I thought, hey, this might be fun, knit a couple of scarfs and give them to my friends as Christmas gifts, you never know. I tried it for 2 weeks. I found myself dreading the day that knitting club was happening. I stuffed my yarn and knitting sticks in the back of the closet and just wanted to forget all about the whole thing. I learned very quickly that knitting was just not for me, it was not a piece of the puzzle of ME, what makes me come alive and what best expresses my authentic self.

I also remember the day that I tried Lindy Hop dancing. Prior to Lindy Hop, I had done salsa dancing since I loved the Latin culture, however, I never fell in *love* with salsa dancing. It felt slightly awkward and sweaty as men that I didn't know came a little too close for comfort breathing into my neck as they groped my body. But the day that I tried Lindy Hop dancing and felt the energy in the room, I was hooked. I became addicted to Lindy Hop dancing. In fact, the first year that I started Lindy Hop dancing, I went out 3-4 nights a week to dance. I loved the intensity, the creativity and the energy of the dance. After dancing, I felt alive, joyous and free. All of my overthinking, overanalyzing and paralyzing emotions would just stop as I focused my energy around the movement of the dance. I started to meet some of my best friends in the Lindy Hop crowd and felt at home with a community that shared similar values and perspectives on life. It was something that I could pour my heart and energy into, and reap so many benefits. I had found another piece of my identity and it would be something that I would go back to over and over again in my life; I was made for Lindy Hop dancing.

There have been so many moments and seasons where I remember finding a piece of my identity. Many times, it seemed that I would find a piece of myself after a major loss, which I call the "crisis of identity." In these seasons of a crisis of identity, it would feel like part of me was dying, and then I would find something that would make me come alive again. For example, when I broke up with my first boyfriend and first love, I felt like part of me was dying. In the midst of the death of part of my soul, I found holistic medicine and became passionate about holistic healing. When my friend Sherry died of cancer, I grieved immensely but birthed my identity in the cancer field and found the greatest calling of my life.

When my son, Noble Thomas died, I felt like my arm had been amputated off of my body and that I would never feel whole again, but I received the gift of Cancer Peace University, what my practice is today, and saw my work with cancer patients be forever transformed. The collateral beauty that comes from tragedy is an experience that is mysterious and defies human logic. But if we can open our hearts to receive it, we can receive our greatest puzzle pieces to our identity amidst our darkest days.

Thus, a profound, internal transformation is something that affects the very core of who you are, your identity. Healing our identity can be a part of healing our souls and our bodies. Many times, people with cancer who experience spontaneous remission find a completely new version of themselves. Part of finding a new identity may be letting go of our negative self-perceptions from experiences in childhood, and healing the wounds of our past. In fact, researchers found that chronic stress from negative self-perceptions wears down the hippocampus in the brain.[1] This is the sea-horse shaped part of your brain that is responsible for memories, emotions and even the beating of your heart.

Thus, our identity and self-perception impacts how much stress we carry and how stress impacts our biology. Researchers found something interesting about perception and stress in the Whitehall study. In fact, researchers found that it is not the objective stress in someone's life that impacts whether or not stress causes a disease process, it is the perception of stress and how the stress is carried based upon the identity of the person. Whitehall and his researchers followed 18,000 men who were 20-64 years old for 10 years to understand the dynamics between stress and heart disease in the lives of these men.[2] The study found the exact opposite of what they expected: those who were the CEOs and executives in the British Civil Service had much lower rates of heart disease than the civil servants. In fact, the lower-class workers had more than twice the rate of heart disease as the upper-class workers. Researchers discovered that it was not the amount of stress upon a worker, but how the stress was perceived based upon the person's self-esteem and self-perception. For those who perceived themselves as less than another person, stress levels increased dramatically compared to workers who had a healthy sense of self.

At this point, you may be asking, how do you develop a healthy sense of self? There are various ways that you can explore and develop your identity including: traveling, going to school, trying something new, learning a new language, learning a new sport or dance, journaling, deepening a spiritual or religious practice or asking friends or family what makes you different or unique. Sometimes, your identity comes out of a gifting, something you naturally excel at that cause others to take notice.

When I first went to college at Vanderbilt University, I was pre-med and thought that I was going to become a medical doctor. In high school, I had LOVED my chemistry classes, calculus classes and science classes. All of a sudden, in college, I completely lost my passion for chemistry. I found myself hating my chemistry lab and chemistry class. At the same time that I despised chemistry labs, my friends kept on saying to me, "you are the best listener that I have ever met." I kept hearing the same thing over and over again about my gift for listening. It struck a chord in me every time someone acknowledged my ability to listen and show empathy. At some point in the process of discovering my identity, I started to think that I would want to pursue counseling.

I found out about the 5-year Master's program in Human Development Counseling at Vanderbilt University and signed up for the classes in the second semester of my freshman year. I found my new classes so fascinating that I decided to drop out of pre-med. In the beginning, it can feel cloudy or unclear, but as you listen to the message that is coming to you through your natural desires and your natural gifting, you will find a true extension of yourself in your career path.

Thus, part of our identity is what we are naturally good at and what we have a natural inclination towards. Also, part of our identity seems to be a blueprint for our wiring that we can discover or reject. Some people describe it as our purpose or destiny on earth. It seems that we can find our purpose, bit by bit, and when we are ready for the next stage. I didn't know that I was going to work with cancer patients when I started my Master's program in counseling. I just knew that I had a gift for listening to people, and I found purpose in helping people process the deep, painful parts of their lives. The purpose of working with cancer patients came many years later.

After graduating from college and working for a few years, I found myself back in my home state, Minnesota. I studied holistic nutrition to become a Nutritional Therapist and started to work with children diagnosed with autism and their families using ABA therapy and nutritional approaches. I thought that autism was my purpose as a Nutritional Therapist. At the same time I was building my practice, I started to connect with a local CSA to get healthy, sustainable food from local farmers. I became friends with the woman who ran the CSA. One day, I emailed her to tell her that my car was vandalized and I didn't know if I could pick up the food that day. She emailed back to say that she had just been diagnosed with breast cancer. I was shocked. I never had a friend receive a cancer diagnosis up until this moment, and I didn't know what to say or what to do.

I remember feeling a strong urge to connect in a deeper way with my friend to support her through her diagnosis. I thought about her a lot and I was drawn to help her in every way that I could. One day, Sherry (I changed her name for the purpose of this book) called to tell me that she was starting to work with a holistic cancer doctor and she wanted me to join her in her appointments. I felt an urgency and even excitement to attend these appointments with her, something I didn't understand at the time. Who gets excited to go to an oncology appointment with a friend? Most people would feel fear and even dread. My excitement and passion seemed odd at the time. Looking back on the path to my purpose, it makes perfect sense now.

When I went with Sherry to her first appointment with the holistic doctor, I saw a quote on the door of the clinic that jumped out at me, "Find peace to your past, purpose to your present and hope for your future." I felt in that moment that my future self was reaching back to me saying: "This is the path to your future." I caught that moment and imprinted it in my mind. In the future, I would remember that clarifying moment as it carried me through my studies in oncology nutrition and my final decision to walk away from autism, and fully commit to supporting cancer patients in my practice.

It became a norm for me to go with Sherry to her appointments, and she started to go to church with me. Our lives became intertwined in many ways. I became familiar with her family, her friends and her children. I remember bits and pieces of our conversation as we walked through her garden one day: "Look at my garden, the storm came last night and just blew it up. It feels like a perfect metaphor for my life right now. My ex is trying to take custody of my son in the middle of my battle with cancer, I mean who does that? And I just found out that the cancer moved from my right breast to my left breast. I'm doing everything that I know to do, but I am just drowning. And now this; my garden is a mess. I just don't know what to do." Sherry seethed with anger and bitterness. I simply listened and let her process her emotional turmoil. I couldn't imagine how difficult her life was at that moment in time. She just needed a compassionate, listening ear.

"I'm so sorry that you are going through all of this, Sherry. I wish there was more that I could do for you. But I am here for you, I am praying for you and I will help in any way that I can." My words escaped my lips and a heavy weight of helplessness came over my soul. It felt like watching an impending car crash from the side of the road without any ability to warn, stop or help those who were about to crash.

One of the most memorable times with my friend, Sherry, came when I found out that she did not know how to have a Christmas for her children. I talked to my dad and we decided to give Sherry and her children the most memorable Christmas of their lives. My friend and I drove to pick Sherry up and her whole mood and countenance changed. "Thank your dad for me, from the bottom of my heart. He did not have to do this. But I'm so thankful. I want to make this Christmas special."

That day we went to several stores and got all of the gifts that her children wanted, food for their Christmas meal, and a beautiful Christmas tree to put in the center of their living room. I remember several moments from that day, but the thing that stands out most in my mind was watching Sherry use one of the motorized carts to navigate through the store. Her breathing was extra labored and she was tired, more tired than usual. At the time, I thought, "She will regain her strength after the New Year and when the Christmas season dies down."

One week after Christmas, I awoke, startled, after a terribly ominous dream about Sherry. We were in a house and there was writing on a wall that looked like calligraphy writing from centuries ago that I couldn't quite decipher. The writing seemed to have a hidden meaning that mocked me. I saw Sherry in the room and I felt a foreboding, dark presence in the room. I tried to get to Sherry, but I could not reach her when all of a sudden, I woke up in a cold, damp sweat. Something is wrong with Sherry, I thought in my head. Two days later, I felt compelled to go see Sherry, but there was an intense snowstorm that swept through all of Minnesota making it treacherous to get anywhere. I didn't heed the compulsion to go to Sherry as a result of the storm. The next morning, I got a call from her son, too early to feel normal. I felt uneasy and I knew something was wrong. "It's mom. She's in the hospital. She asked me to call you to have you come." He urgently uttered the words that I didn't want to hear, but I should have known were coming.

I rushed as fast as I could to the hospital and found Sherry to be very weak. Her voice was soft and faint. We talked urgently. Everything felt so fragile, like if I would breathe wrong the ceiling would come crashing down around us. Feeling helpless again, I listened as Sherry told me what happened: "I started vomiting blood late last night and my son had to rush me to the hospital. He doesn't even have his license, but I couldn't drive myself. My doctor says my liver is failing." She couldn't share much more than that as she had already expended all of her energy. Her family was coming soon to talk to her and the doctor. Doing all I could do, I left in a state of shock, remorse and helplessness.

I decided I would come every day and give the family some space to talk to the doctor today. The next time I saw Sherry she was in a semi-comatose state and couldn't communicate at all. I regretted not saying more the first time I saw her.

After that day, Sherry was transferred to hospice care. I fought tooth and nail to get her out of there. I knew that she desperately wanted to live. Her children were still young and two of her children had special needs. She was terrified of what would happen to them if she died. I was there every day, 7 days straight for almost 8 hours a day. Eventually, I was kicked out of the hospice center because I was too vocal, advocating for Sherry's rights. When I asked her, "Sherry, do you want water? Are you thirsty?" Sherry would nod her head, yes, as she was too weak to speak.

The hospice care team explained to me, in a condescending way, that "Sherry doesn't need water right now. In fact, it is better for us to not give her water because when she dies, she will feel euphoric." Some sort of bullshit line like that was fed to me. I didn't buy it. In my mind, it was simple: I ask her if she wants water, she nods her head, yes, give her water. These hospice people sounded insane to me. In fact, I called a lawyer to explore my options in this situation. The lawyer was as shocked and enraged as I was. If someone nods their head yes in response to a question because they are too weak to speak, then it is in their rights to receive what they desire. In Sherry's case, she wanted water. It was absolutely illegal what was happening in front of my eyes, but I needed Sherry to sign me over to be the power of attorney so that I could have a legally binding voice. I was the only person spending enough time with her to discover the subtle moments that she was cognizant and able to respond by nodding her head and giving small gestures or facial expressions. Everyone else just assumed that she was completely non-responsive because they would come in and out in less than 5 minutes without engaging her in those subtle ways. We attempted to sign over the power of attorney to me, but our attempt failed. The staff manipulated her family to take me off of the list of visitors because of their fear of being sued.

The day after I was kicked out of the hospice care center, I left my house and drove to the hospice care center like every other day that week. I operated on complete autopilot. I imagined myself breaking into the hospice center and kidnapping Sherry. I imagined all sorts of insane ways of dealing with the situation at hand, but then I just found myself sitting in my car before the sunrise like a complete idiot, trying to figure out a disguise to get into the hospice center. I went to the door and tried to pretend to be a visitor for Sherry's roommate, except I couldn't remember her name. I tried to explain what she looked like as I tried to hide my face behind a hat. They quickly figured out it was me, the woman who had been kicked out the day previously. I left, but felt completely lost and livid at the same time. Cursing, I said to myself, "I'm going to sue these insane idiots for withholding water from my friend. I can't believe that they are so inhumane here." I imagined all kinds of acts of revenge, but the main one that I settled on was to write the most god-awful review on Google that I could think of to warn families to stay away from this complete hellhole.

I remember going to see clients that day and felt like I was out of my body and couldn't find any train of thought. My mind was fragmented and confused. The next morning, I got the call that Sherry had died. Part of me felt like it died with her. And for many months after her death, I grieved and felt waves of depression, anger and hopelessness.

In the end, I felt honored to be a small part of Sherry's journey. I had faced death and survived. And I was starting to learn more about how to integrate my experience of living with the reality of mortality. This experience became imprinted in my soul, and I found myself reading every book I could read about cancer. My calling to work with cancer patients was stirred within my soul during every conversation and interaction that I had with Sherry during her diagnosis.

Finding our authentic self can be painful as we delve into the most intimate and vulnerable moments that life offers. For me, being with Sherry in hospice care center and staring death in the face was the most intense experience in my life up until that point. The experience was complex, devastating and beautiful all at the same time. I couldn't have thought of anything more meaningful than what I shared with Sherry. Sherry also left me with the greatest gift any human can give: she gave me the gift of finding a huge piece of my identity. Working with people with cancer has become a natural extension of who I am. The times that I find myself feeling the most alive are always after my one-on-one sessions with cancer patients.

Interestingly enough, becoming self-actualized has been found to impact longevity. Norman Shealy, a neurosurgeon, studied 4 different groups of people and found many insights into how internal dispositions affect the development of disease in the body.[3] Participants in Group 1 of the study identified as having a hopeless outlook on life. Those in Group 2 operated out of a lifelong pattern of blame or anger. Participants in Group 3 bounced between hopelessness and anger, whereas those in Group 4 were self-actualized and believed that **"happiness is an inside job."**

Throughout his research, Shealy found that 75% of those who die of heart disease and 15% of those who die of cancer fall into the category of anger and blame. Those who found themselves in the hopeless category die 35 years younger than Group 4, those who identified as being self-actualized. Further, those with a hopeless disposition were found to die 75% of the time of cancer and 15% of the time of heart disease. **Hopelessness is truly dangerous to your health, whereas pursuing and becoming self-actualized may be one of the secrets to longevity.**

Most cancer treatments treat the physical symptom, the tumor or cancer itself, and completely overlook the underlying causes of the cancer. Nearly all reported cases of cancer miracles documented report that the cancer survivor has made dramatic changes to their whole life. They have changed their diet and their lifestyle, they have removed all stress from their lives and most importantly they have healed their internal emotional stress, which is the primary cause of cancer.

Cancer is a physical symptom of prolonged internal emotional stress. Although most people endure stress and trauma during their life, it is the way we handle the stress that determines if we get cancer, whether we repress our feelings and internalize the stress or not. This may sound unreal to some. But, when you know how stress causes cancer, then and only then can you have the confidence to make the necessary changes and reverse cancer within your body.

"Cancer is a message to you from your body. It is communicating to you that something is not right within you, emotionally. Cancer is not a death-sentence, it is an opportunity to heal within."[4]

For those who have not discovered cancer from this perspective, this quote may seem unbelievable. However, case after case of spontaneous remission demonstrates that the person who went into remission, without the expectation of their oncologist, dealt with major emotional roots to their diagnosis and reworked their entire life to make stress minimal or manageable.

There have been many studies done to try to understand what types of personality traits can cause someone to be more susceptible to develop different types of diseases. Personality traits and character traits can cause people to internalize stress more readily and play a role into a diagnosis of a disease condition. Let's explore a few of these studies to help us understand that cancer is no different than other disease states.

First, let's look at stomach ulcers and personality traits. Researchers at Finnish Institute of Occupational Health studied more than 4,000 people and found that those with impulsive personality traits were 2.4 times more likely to develop stomach ulcers.[5] The reasoning behind this data is that people who act more impulsively tend to respond to stress with a higher production of stomach acid, triggering ulcers.

Further, people who have anxiety disorders are more likely to be treated for high blood pressure.[6] In fact, a study from Northern Arizona University found that an increased production of stress hormones from anxiety elevated blood pressure.[7]

In addition, researchers at Ohio State University created small wounds on the arms of healthy people to watch how these wounds healed depending on their emotional disposition.[8] Those who were found to be angry healed much slower than those who remained calm. After four days, 30% of the angry patients healed their wounds whereas 70% of patients who were calm healed their wounds.

Interestingly enough, research has found that optimistic people live an average of 7.5 years longer than those who are pessimistic.[9] In addition, researchers found that optimism boosts the immune system.[10] Again, I have Sjhira to thank for helping me shift from a negative state of mind to a more positive state of mind, which most likely added years to my life! Thank you, Sjhira! I hope that you also find your Sjhira to help you shift to a place of optimism!

As you can see, there are many different personality traits and emotional dispositions that have been correlated to a variety of conditions. Stress plays a large role in this, as different ways of thinking, behaving, and feeling contribute to how we handle or do not handle stress in our lives. Now, we will dive into emotional dispositions and personality traits connected with the development of cancer.

Lawrence LeShan, MD, first described what became known as the carcinogenic personality in the following manner: someone who begins life feeling incomplete, empty and powerless to do anything about it. As an adult, this personality type tries to fill their emptiness with belonging, status or power. What LeShan found with his cancer patients, was that when his patients lost their external source of wholeness through death, retirement, the loss of a job, finances, etc., six months or so later, they were diagnosed with cancer.[11]

One of the largest and most in depth studies on emotional coping skills and cancer compares emotional reactions of malignant melanoma patients with cardiovascular patients. In 1984, Lydia Temoshok and her team measured the physiological responses to stressful stimuli in 3 distinct groups: patients with malignant melanoma, patients with heart disease and the control group, which had no diagnosed disease. This study found that cancer patients tend to experience emotional stressors with measurable physical effects on their system while managing to suppress the awareness of these feelings.

The Type C Personality as defined by the results of this 1984 study found that people who develop cancer tend to be cooperative, patient, passive, accepting and lacking assertiveness. Those with The Type C Personality tend to avoid conflict out of a desire to be liked and a desire to please people. Instead of expressing emotions, The Type C Personality has learned to repress their emotions and lack the assertiveness to get their needs met in relationships.[12]

During the study, each participant was connected to a dermograph, a device that records the body's electrical reactions in the skin, while they were exposed to slides with insulting phrases like "You are ugly" or "You have only yourself to blame."[13] After reading the slide, participants recorded how they felt in that moment. The researchers were able to compare the participant's subjective response with an objective reading from the dermograph. The participants with melanoma were found to deny any awareness that the messages on the slides provoked an emotional response. In fact, they would record that they felt fine with the message on the slide at the same time that the dermograph showed nervous system distress. Further, those with The Type C Personality were found to not be consciously aware of their habitual suppression of emotions.

Other studies about emotional processing habits and cancer have confirmed the findings from the 1984 Temoshok study. In fact, a study performed in Melbourne, Australia with over 600 colorectal cancer patients found that those with cancer were more likely to demonstrate emotional processing habits of denial and repression of anger. Further, the cancer patients in this study were found to suppress emotional reactions to avoid conflict in relationships.[14]

I still remember a conversation that I had with a client diagnosed with ovarian cancer. She said, "We went to the cabin this weekend and after dinner, everyone went off to the lake and left me by myself to clean up. I thought about how when I was growing up in such a large family, I was overlooked many times. I would clean the kitchen, cook and help with the household. One night, I came home from school and my mom had a huge plate of food for my brother saved, but I was left to make my own food." Her voice was sad, lonely and shaky.

She went on, this time, her emotions pointed towards her husband, "My husband bought a brand-new race car without telling me. I still haven't gotten over that one." My client recounted situation after situation that left her feeling overlooked, lonely and unimportant. Understand this, her childhood wasn't abusive or traumatic in a massive scale; however, small moments of feeling overlooked, emotionally neglected and insignificant led her to have a low self-esteem and a negative perception of herself as an adult. She also had a tendency of repressing her emotions to avoid conflict.

When emotions are suppressed, the immune system becomes suppressed as a result. Dr. Robert Ader coined the phrase psychoneuroimmunology, which is the study of how our psychology impacts our immune system. Neuropeptides are brain chemicals of mood and behavior, which communicate to the immune system.[15] As a result, we have bits of our brain floating everywhere, in constant communication with our biology. Immune cells have neuro-receptor sites to receive neuropeptides from the brain, which will either stimulate or repress the immune system. Also, neuropeptides can signal to cancer cells to cause them to grow or travel. Our mind is a constant flow of information as it moves along cells, organs and systems of the body, mostly unconsciously, in order to link and coordinate major systems of the body for better or for worse.

Another expert in the arena of emotional processing habits, trauma and cancer is the German oncologist Dr. Hamer. Prior to approaching cancer as an unresolved emotional trauma or conflict, Dr. Hamer had worked with cancer patients using traditional oncology treatments. However, when he was diagnosed with testicular cancer himself, he began to question many aspects of the approach to treating cancer by focusing only on the shrinking or removal of the tumor. Dr. Hamer was diagnosed with testicular cancer only 2 short months after his son, Dirk, was murdered. He knew intuitively that he had developed cancer as a direct result of the emotional trauma involved with the death of his son. He began to ask deeper questions to his oncology patients, going on to find that nearly all of his oncology patients could point to an unresolved emotional trauma that may be connected to their cancer diagnosis.

Through a process of many years, Dr. Hamer developed an approach to cancer called German New Medicine to focus on the unresolved trauma of cancer patients. Through his work, Dr. Hamer found that many cancer patients were unable to share their thoughts, emotions, fears and joys with other people. He coined the phrase "psycho-emotional isolation" to describe the phenomenon of his cancer patients' inability to emotionally connect with others. He found cancer patients to not only be isolated from others emotionally, but also to be isolated from themselves; not understanding, connecting with or expressing their deepest emotions.

It's not that people without cancer don't go through trauma and emotional pain, it is the fact that there is a healthy process of grieving and moving through trauma that results in good physical health and an unhealthy way of getting stuck in trauma that can result in a disease process.

A conversation with one of my clients reminds me of the phrase psycho-emotional isolation that Dr. Hamer coined. "My whole life is a series of traumatic events. If cancer is unresolved emotional trauma, then we need to revisit my entire life." My client, clearly exacerbated by the discovery that cancer stems from unresolved emotional trauma, didn't even know how to begin. Most of her relationships ended as quickly as they began, as she couldn't figure out how to develop intimate bonds. She grew up with a mother who had debilitating MS. Thus, she couldn't properly care for her children. My client, as a result, ran away from home when she was 15 years old. She couldn't remember a healthy relationship with a woman or a man in her life.

Identifying trauma is the first step in resolving trauma as I have worked with clients who simply cannot recognize any negative experiences in their lives. This is the worst case scenario of psychological suppression that can only be shifted by a person coming out of denial and control into a place of openness and curious discovery.

Now, I want to point you to the companion workbook to address your own trauma and come out of a place of denial into a place of openness and emotional discovery that will lead to freedom and healing.

Section 1: Getting Right with Me

Chapter 5: Digging Deeper

My heart beating out of my chest, and my thoughts racing, I couldn't breathe and sleep evaded me. I tried to find a comfortable position to lie down and find rest, but the task proved to be impossible. What was happening to me? I couldn't understand why I was experiencing these episodes at night. Previously, I never struggled to find sleep. Now, it was a different story. There was something wrong, but I couldn't put my finger on exactly what it was; just the humming noise of something I couldn't quite decipher.

I never thought I was an anxious person, until I met Mary Elizabeth Byrd or "MeBird." The essence of peace, MeBird carried herself with such grace, you would have thought she was floating on a cloud. When I was getting to know her, I would watch her reactions to things that would cause me stress and I was baffled when she would calmly handle pressure coming from every side of her life. Where did she find this peace and emotional stability?

Every night, I started finding someone to talk to before I went to bed to ease the panic that would erupt first in my endless thoughts, then in my racing heart and finally, in the loss of my breath. If I could talk through the thoughts that seemed to be all over the place, without a common thread to weave them together, then eventually my heart would slow down, my breath would come back and I could find sleep.

Prior to college, I didn't even know what a "panic attack" was. But here I was, night after tormenting night, finding strategies to navigate the underlying anxiety that plagued my soul. Clearly, there was something wrong. But beyond the anxiety, what was it? What was causing such angst within me?

The root causes to my anxiety would take years to uncover, but meeting MeBird set me on a path to discover what peace she carried that evaded me at that time. I soon realized that the beginning stages of unraveling my anxiety started with off-loading my racing thoughts on a daily basis. I began the habit of journaling again. I had kept diaries when I was much younger, but I would write things like: "I think that I like Jeremy, but I'm too scared to talk to him." The thoughts of an 8-year-old were much different than the thoughts of an 18-year-old, yet I longed for the simplicity of my youth.

I think I may have made Starbucks rich with my daily habit of buying a "chai tea latte with soy milk no water," finding a plushy chair and listening to Enya on my CD player while I dumped all of my thoughts into my journal. Eventually, after I dumped enough of my jumbled-up thoughts, up would pop an emotion in which I was completely unaware and I would be sitting in my plushy, purple chair sobbing for the whole Starbucks world to see. I didn't care, I felt like I was making progress! I was releasing deep emotions for the first time! After releasing these emotions, I would feel significantly more centered and less anxious.

I finally was taking the time to get to know myself, to understand my thoughts and to grow in emotional intelligence. I was developing self-awareness and digging deep to find the emotions underneath the constant buzz of anxiety. Many times, people with cancer just scratch the surface of potential emotional root causes correlated to their diagnosis and don't fully resolve their most disappointing and traumatic experiences. In fact, I remember one such client.

Susan (I changed her name for the purpose of this book) came to me after a second diagnosis of breast cancer, just 9 short months after her treatments from her first diagnosis finished. She called me and said, "This time, I want to approach my diagnosis very differently. The first time I was diagnosed, I was in shock and terrified. I felt like a robot, just going through the motions. As a result, I just submitted to the doctor, doing everything he said to do and nothing outside of what he was prescribing. It wasn't until my treatments were over that I cried and started to catch up to the reality of my diagnosis. My mom was diagnosed with cancer when I was still a teenager and she died several years later. As a result, I have carried a lot of sadness in my life. I want to be involved and proactive during my diagnosis this time and I want to do what I can to heal myself."

At first, I thought that we were on track to see some progress on the emotional side of things. However, as Susan and I began the program, she became very fixated on the physical parts of the protocol, making sure she was juicing 3 times a day, doing a sauna, enema and rebounding every day. She was making gourmet vegetarian meals and most of her time was spent in the kitchen. I remember a conversation that I had with her that struck me at the time, "When I do something, I don't just do it, I become obsessed and take it to the extreme. For example, I didn't just attend yoga classes to exercise, I decided to become an instructor. When I began spinning, I went through the process to become a spinning instructor. It's never enough for me to have a hobby or do something that makes me feel good. I have to be the best in order to feel good about myself." Susan seemed to approach her holistic support with cancer in that same manner. She quickly became a model client, doing everything I suggested and more.

However, when we would try to dive deeper on the emotional side, it never felt like we could sync and uncover the deeper roots. She didn't outwardly express any emotions and was a very internal person. When she spoke about things in the past that bothered her, she spoke monotone and very matter-of-fact. She never had a moment of emotional release or revelation of the cause of cancer on the emotional side, nor did she implement a daily practice of delving into the deeper side. She was either too busy making gourmet vegetarian food, didn't believe that the emotional side mattered or she couldn't allow herself to dive into the emotional pain and chaos that held her captive for so long.

What I have found in my practice is that there is a difference between acknowledging the root emotional and relational causes to cancer on the surface level and finding the closure and resolve necessary for a profound, internal transformation to occur in the body. Susan, along with many other clients, come to me thinking that they can eat, supplement and use holistic cancer therapies to find healing and resolve to their cancer, without addressing the trauma, internal emotional processing habits and relational conflicts that continuously imprint upon their biology.

In this chapter, Digging Deep, we will dissect a major study that explores the effects of self- help strategies and group counseling on the survival outcomes of cancer patients. In fact, there have been multiple studies on group counseling and the impact to the prognosis of a cancer diagnosis. However, the studies seem to conflict with one another, until we look at a study that brings clarity. This study is called The Cunningham Study and it sheds light to why studies examining how self-help strategies impact survival outcomes with cancer seemingly contradict each other.

In the 1990s, Cunningham performed a study with The University of Toronto for 47 people diagnosed with Stage III Colon Cancer having a 30% chance of survival. Initially, it seemed that group therapy failed to have an impact on survival outcomes.[1] However, a small percentage of people had significant improvement after therapy with 7 women living significantly longer than the others and 2 of 7 still alive 8 years after the start of the study. The number is too small to be statistically significant, but Cunningham took time to review the 7 people and the 2 that were still alive and found that a person's level of involvement in the therapy had a major impact on survival outcomes.

The 7 survivors sought other approaches to healing in addition to the group therapy and spent time meditating, journaling, writing intentional gratitude's in addition to changing daily habits and routines. Cunningham found the 7 women to have a "get up and go attitude." The results of this study prompted Cunningham to do another study to look at highly motivated patients who had an interest in self-help. Thus, in 2002, Cunningham did a qualitative analysis of the actual process of psychotherapy and self-help techniques in patients with metastatic cancer.[2] There was 100 hours devoted to the study of each participant to find out the details of their approach and their level of involvement. There were 9 patients found to be highly involved who devoted regular daily time to meditating, visualization, cognitive monitoring, journaling and relaxation activities among other self-help strategies. Seven of the 9 had a high-quality life and lived 2 years past their prognosis. Two of the 9 had complete and unexpected spontaneous remissions, which lasted years after this study. There were 8 participants who were less involved than average and were unconvinced that self-help would change their disease outcomes or felt unworthy of the efforts. These 8 participants also did not have a good quality of life, had low self-esteem and only 1 lived 2 years past their prognosis.

Overall, the participants who were highly involved in self-help therapies lived 3 times longer than those with low involvement. Now, this is significant! Look at the charts below to see conditions associated with poor survival outcomes and longer survival outcomes to understand further what this study discovered:

Conditions associated with poor survival outcomes:

- Inflexibility associated with low self-esteem or fixed worldview
- Skepticism about self-help techniques or a limited ability to apply them
- Other activities seemed more immediately appealing
- Meaning was habitually sought outside the individual from some external source
- Strong, contrary views about the validity of spiritual ideas

Conditions associate with longer survival outcomes:

- Strong will to live
- Actual changes in habits of thought and activity
- Relaxation practices, meditation, mental imaging, cognitive monitoring
- Becoming involved in a search for meaning in one's life

In conclusion, how deeply a cancer patient engages and believes in the process of healing and using self-help strategies matters in terms of impacting survival outcomes. How deep and involved are you willing to go to reach the psychological roots of your diagnosis?

I have had clients completely avoid exploring emotional roots to their diagnosis and I have had clients who have gone as deep as they can to resolve past negative experiences and trauma. My clients who go the deepest on the emotional and spiritual side tend to have the most benefits and the most progress. For example, I started working with a client diagnosed with uterine cancer named Stephanie (I changed her name for the purpose of this book).

I can still feel the ambience of the room as I received a call from Stephanie. She urgently shared with me, "I was told to call you, I was recently diagnosed with uterine cancer and I don't know what to do. I am trying to avoid surgery as I am so young. I don't know how this could've happened to me. I eat organic, exercise, don't eat sugar or drink coffee and I even studied nutrition because I am so passionate about healthy living. I am the healthiest of my friends and family, except for this cancer diagnosis. Can you help me?"

I listened carefully to her story and felt a lot of compassion for her. She was in her 40s and had 2 young children, too young to be diagnosed with cancer. I suspected that she had an unresolved emotional trauma since her lifestyle was already so clean and healthy. "I can definitely help. My client with prostate cancer went from a 134 on the PSA test to 1.3 in just 8 weeks. If you already have such a healthy lifestyle, we may want to explore some potential emotional or relational triggers in our sessions." I explained and emphasized my enthusiasm to help Stephanie. Newly niched in cancer, I was eager to take on her case. She was warm and open, and it seemed like we would quickly make progress.

When Stephanie came in for our first session, I asked many questions about her past and health history. Through asking her more detailed questions, I found some answers. I asked her, "What is the most traumatic thing that you have experienced in your life?" She said, "I was date raped when I was 17 years old, but that was a long time ago. I think I resolved it." I asked her if she could tell me more about what happened, curious to see if this was the emotional root of her diagnosis. Date rape can be very challenging to resolve.

Stephanie elaborated on the most intense trauma in her life, "I was only 17 years old and was dating my first boyfriend. I was so excited to finally be in a relationship after years of watching my friends date. I was a hopeless romantic at that time in my life and thought that I would be swept away by my prince. Instead, I was rudely awakened to the reality that men are dogs and that all they want is sex. One night, in my boyfriend's truck, he pushed me to go further than I wanted to go physically. I said over and over again "No, no, no, please stop." All of a sudden, he pushed past my intended boundaries and forced himself on top of me. I just froze inside and couldn't breathe. I focused on a tree outside of the truck until it was over. As soon as he was done, I quietly asked to go home. At home, I fell, crumpled in a ball on my bed, sobbing at the loss of my innocence." She continued to share that she had thought it was over. In fact, she went on to marry, have children and rarely thought about the trauma from her past.

I asked her to picture her ex-boyfriend and tell me how she felt. As Stephanie closed her eyes to reflect on her ex-boyfriend, her voice got shaky. "Wait a minute, I am getting hot all over and I feel this intense anger boiling up in me." Stephanie, looking confused, tapped into emotions that she had not felt except for right after the incident. The strong emotions connected to the trauma revealed the opposite of what her conscious mind believed, the deep wound was still festering in her soul and manifested within her uterus.

When Stephanie went through her experience of date rape, she didn't really have anyone to talk to. Her parents forbade her from dating and didn't like her boyfriend, so she couldn't open up to them. She didn't want him to get in trouble or get arrested, as she did like him, so she didn't tell any of her teachers. She also felt like it was partly her fault as they had been pushing physical boundaries for a while and she grew up in a party town where one-night stands were part of the norm.

Through the process of several sessions, Stephanie and I redesigned the memories of all her past sexual relationships. She went home after one of our sessions and threw up several times. Stephanie really dug deep to feel all of the feelings she had repressed at the time.

As we explored the memory in one session, I asked Stephanie, "What do you wish you would have said to your ex-boyfriend that you never had the chance to say? Stay in the memory, face your ex and say exactly what you have wanted to say all these years." Stephanie took a deep breath, closed her eyes and stammered, "Jeff, you were my first boyfriend and I thought that I was in love with you. I trusted you completely. I grew up watching fairy tales of princesses falling in love with princes. I was so excited to finally be living a romance of my own. When you betrayed me, and took my innocence from me, I felt broken-hearted for the first time in my life. Fantasies surrounding romance were destroyed forever in one moment. You were selfish, evil and have no idea how much torment you put me through. I felt nothing, completely numb for months on end, and then I would feel rage and intense hatred towards my sexuality and myself. It would take me years to open up and be in a relationship again, with my now husband. I have hated you for years. And I even hated myself for years."

Tears streaming down her face, Stephanie opened her eyes and looked at me, emotions as fresh as when the trauma first happened. Timidly, Stephanie said, "I didn't know that was all still in me."

I paused for a moment, and then I said, "Do you feel ready to forgive Jeff?" Stephanie looked down and thought for a moment. I softly continued, "Forgiveness is not about Jeff, it's about finding peace for your own soul and moving past what happened so that you don't have to live with the hatred and anger towards Jeff."

Stephanie nodded and said, "Yes, I want to forgive and move on."

I led Stephanie in a simple forgiveness exercise towards Jeff, "Look at Jeff in the memory and say these words and anything else that comes to you, 'Jeff, today I choose to forgive you, not because you apologized or because you deserve it. I choose to forgive you because my soul needs peace.'"

After the moment lingered and dissipated, I looked at Stephanie and said the following, "Can we look at the memory again? Can you close your eyes, walk through the memory and see what is still lingering?" Stephanie closed her eyes and looked. And then I said the following, "Now, I want you to open your heart as I invite God to come into that memory with you and heal you. God, will you come into this memory with Stephanie and show her what you want to show her?"

I waited with Stephanie. After a minute or two, Stephanie opened her eyes, glistening with tears and said, "I feel peace. It's gone. I can't really see the memory anymore. I don't feel any of the emotions that I did either." Relieved, Stephanie took a deep breath out. It would be a few weeks before I heard from Stephanie again. She sent me an email, short and sweet but full of excitement, "I had a scan done and they couldn't find any cancer in my uterus!"

We connected on a call that week and Stephanie was astonished at the spontaneous healing as she laughed, "The doctors didn't know what to say, but we canceled the surgery." Stephanie postponed the surgery because she didn't want a hysterectomy, and wanted time to discover how cancer developed in her body.

In the end, her cancer regressed with no need for surgery because of her ability to deeply address and release the trauma that she experienced when she was date raped at 17.

Another exercise besides redesigning memories that I find helpful for my clients to dig deeper is journaling. I feel myself losing some men reading my book right now; before you give up on me and decide that this is not for you, hear me out. Journaling does not have to mean what you think it means! I know that many of you are thinking, "I don't know what to write or it makes me feel uncomfortable. I'm not a touchy, feely person. So…I'm not going to go there!" Wait: there are options! Some people do better talking to themselves and recording their own voices on their iPhones, especially if you are an extrovert and an auditory learner. There are many forms and fashions for journaling and the benefits are tremendous.

A huge component to healing and to a profound, internal transformation is awareness and emotional intelligence. Journaling is a way to grow in both awareness and emotional intelligence. If you don't know how you feel or it is hard to connect with your emotions and express them to loved ones, journaling will help you overcome the learning curve involved in developing your emotional intelligence. When trauma victims write about their experiences, physiological changes occur in their bodies including increased blood flow and a boost to the immune system. Further, the immune systems of those with cancer were found to be stronger, and the tumors smaller, for those who were in touch with their emotions.[3]

I find that the most helpful way to start journaling is through free-association journaling. This simply means to write down all of your thoughts as the thoughts are coming without judging, editing or blocking them. Just write. As you write, listen to relaxing and meditative music. I like Solfeggio frequencies. The longer you write, the closer you will get to emotional expression.

Follow your thoughts to what you notice in your body. Are you noticing anything in your body like pain in a certain area, increased heart rate, upset stomach, trouble breathing or a desire to cry? If you are, allow yourself to identify the emotion and release it. Soon, you will learn to identify anxiety with an increased heart rate and racing thoughts.

At some point in this process, you may feel like crying or screaming. Allow yourself to feel and express your emotions as they come. If you are better able to express vulnerable emotions by yourself, make sure you find a space without an audience. I felt comfortable crying in Starbucks, as random strangers watching me cry didn't bother me.

The goal with this type of journaling is to connect your thoughts to your emotions and to open yourself up to connect with your subconscious mind, which holds memories. Your memories hold the keys to understanding your belief system and to finding those maladaptive core beliefs that need to shift.

You may gain insight into why you feel the way that you feel. After you express an emotion, just listen or watch your mind space for added insight. You may see an image or a memory flash before your mind. Write down the image or memory. After journaling, meditation is a good strategy to help connect your conscious mind to your subconscious mind. It's time to go into your companion workbook to answer the questions, do the exercises and learn how to meditate.

Section 2: Relationships Reflect Me: What Do You See?

Chapter 1: The Broken Heart

The phone rang, startling me from my deep thoughts. I looked down at the caller ID: Joe. I haven't heard from him in months, I wondered, why is he calling? My thoughts wandered further as I contemplated the last year of our relationship at the same time that I eagerly answered his phone call.

Exactly one-year prior, we were both in L.A. doing an internship. We had been best friends from college and had a "define the relationship" talk prior to moving out to L.A. It didn't go the way that I had imagined that it would. I remember him coming to my house to give me my car back and saying in a quiet, serious tone, "Hey Megan, we need to talk, can we go to Starbucks later?" I could tell by the tone of his voice that it was one of those talks that could either be the best conversation of my life or the absolute worst. I was hoping for the former.

At Starbucks, Joe wasted no time and poured his guts out to me, "I like you, I really like you, but I think that we need to lay down our relationship before we go to L.A."

Who talks like that? I thought to myself as I tried desperately to push that sentence from my mind and act like those words never came forth. Looking down, I could not think of anything profound to say to shift his perspective. In fact, the way the words came out, so decisive, I could tell that he had been thinking about it for a while now, and had come to his conclusion. It also sounded like someone around him had influenced his thinking. It just didn't make sense, and didn't sound like Joe, my best friend. I mean really, lay down the relationship? What does that even mean? And who breaks up with someone before even going on one official date?

One of my childhood besties would point out after our conversation, "Wait, did he just break up with you before you ever dated? I don't think he can even do that. This is just ridiculous." Becca broke me out of my defeated, hopeless posture by giving me a good laugh.

"You're right," I retorted back, "How can he break up with me when we never even dated? This is ridiculous. I mean who does that?" At the same time, I felt my insides dying from sadness.

Back at Starbucks, I tried to pull back tears, but the tears resisted me and began to flow as the weight of his words hit my heart like a brick. I had been patiently waiting for the day that we could openly confess our feelings to one another. For some reason, that day never seemed to come. Five years of being best friends, we just kept playing the role of friends while everyone around us took note of the special bond we had. Secretly, I had told a few of my best friends about my undying love for Joe, as I felt that eventually we would get married. I just never knew when that would be. In college, Joe found out that his dad cheated on his mom and they ended up getting a divorce. I knew that as a result, relationships were complicated for him and he was cautious at best in our relationship.

Snapping myself out of my daydream, I quickly answered the phone call before it dropped, "Hello?" I tried to act casual, but my heart was racing and my voice felt shaky.

"Hey, Megan?" Joe asked in a deep, confident tone.

"Oh, hey Joe, how's it going?" I feigned being relaxed and acted like it was completely normal for him to be calling after not talking for over 6 months.

"Hey, I'm good, I wanted to talk to you. You know, I have been thinking a lot about you and I miss you. I really want to pursue a relationship with you. It took me some time to sort out my life and figure out what I want to do with my life and now I know that I want to go to law school. When we were just graduating from school and doing our internship in L.A., I was so stressed about the uncertainty of it all, and I wasn't confident in what I wanted to do with my life like you were. I felt so much pressure and I was just broke. I couldn't imagine dating you at that time. But, now, I am ready, if you want to try?"

Dramatically, the phone dropped out of my hands and hung up on Joe. Squealing in delight, I shouted across the hallway to Sjhira, my roommate, "It's Joe on the phone, he wants to start dating!" Sjhira bounced into my room shouting in disbelief, "What in the world? Really? Oh my gosh! Call him back!" Sjhira grabbed my pillow and jumped on my bed, intently waiting to hear the rest of the conversation. I quickly called him back, "Sorry, Joe, the phone dropped. Yeah, I think that we can try, if that's what you want?" I again acted casually committed, but inside fireworks were going off. This was *it!* The moment that I had been waiting on for years finally came, after I had completely lost all hope that it would ever happen. I had given up just a few weeks before then and decided that I was going to walk the single road. It had been years that my heart and mind were obsessed with the idea of dating Joe and I could not believe that it was actually happening after so many moments of gut-wrenching disappointment. The conversation before L.A. was actually one of a few conversations that left me completely broken.

I remembered that after our internship, we took a trip to Nashville to see our friends. Stopping in Chicago, we stayed with my friend, Holly, for the night. We went out with Holly and her friends and went home to end up in a fight that completely broke my heart. I remembered him saying, "I just don't feel like dating you." In that moment, he was so callused towards me. I had never experienced this side of Joe. I couldn't even believe those words escaped his lips.

Was this how little he thought of me when I spent every moment of every day thinking about him?

I immediately started sobbing and I couldn't stop as he tried to sleep on the ground next to the couch that I was sleeping on. I think I cried half the night with Joe tossing and turning on the ground. In the morning, my eyes puffy, voice hoarse, I decided that I wasn't going to talk to Joe the entire way to Nashville. Picking up our friend Sjhira in Chicago, we started to drive the 10-hour ride to Nashville. I was stone cold, staring out the window without a word to anyone. Periodically, tears of deep sadness and rejection streamed down my face. No one talked for the entire drive. It was excruciating for me, but I'm sure that it was equally painful for everyone else in the car.

Again, snapping back to reality after taking stock of all of the low moments in my relationship with Joe, I looked at Sjhira after the surprising conversation with Joe and started laughing, "Wow, it's really happening. I cannot believe this!"

Since we had been best friends for many years in college, our relationship became serious very fast and Joe decided to move to Nashville again so that we could be in the same city. I went home for Thanksgiving and helped him move all of his stuff to Nashville, to start over. We had a wonderful few months of dating in Nashville and I had never been so in love and truly happy with life. One of my friends made the comment to me, "Wow, you look more beautiful than ever. Being in love looks good on you."

And then my heart broke again. Within 4 months of our new relationship, I started crying at the end of our dates. I didn't understand it at the time. But, I felt that something was different. Joe emotionally shut down. I couldn't reach him anymore. He had been angry with his father for having an affair and leaving his mother. The bitterness and resentment spread and suffocated all of his emotions. I tried desperately to reach Joe, but he felt like a brick wall.

During a holiday that year, I traveled with my family to Colorado to ski. My mom and I went to have massages one day. It was during the massage that I heard something that changed the path of my life forever. While I was in a deep state of relaxation, I heard the words "If you break up with him, I will heal him. You are a crutch. If you break up with him, I will heal him." I audibly gasped as I heard those words. I couldn't believe what I had just heard and yet I knew that it was true. I couldn't fix Joe and if I was in the way of him getting healed, I needed to get out of the way. Besides, I thought to myself, he will probably get healed and then we can get back together again and have the relationship that I always dreamed we would have.

As soon as I got back from the skiing trip to Colorado, I spent some time with Joe and shared with him what I had heard during the massage. I told him that we needed to take a break on our relationship. Stunned, Joe sat there and stared into space. I tried to comfort him and he pushed me away saying, "You should leave." Tears spontaneously spilled from my eyes as I felt my heart break again. Ironically, I had just broken my own heart.

I cried on and off for months, felt waves of anger and depression as I grieved the loss of my first love and best friend, again. I felt like I could not move on and as if I would never love again. A few months later, I was sitting on the couch and talking to Sjhira. I told Sjhira, "I feel like I'm becoming more normal again, but I just cannot stop thinking that Joe is my husband. I feel stuck."

Sjhira looked at me and mused aloud, "You know, when we were in college? I heard you speaking Spanish to Mirza on the phone one day. As I listened briefly to your conversation, I heard you come alive in a way that I never had previously. I thought to myself, Megan might marry someone from another country." As soon as Sjhira uttered those words, the phrase "Joe is my husband" broke from my brain completely and all of a sudden, I was open to new possibilities. I felt hope instead of hopelessness. In that moment, I believed fully that I would meet someone new, perhaps someone from Latin America?

I would not be the person that I am today without relationships with key people in my life: my mom, my dad, my closest friends, my mentors, my husband and my children. I have been transformed by key relationships as I have allowed my vulnerabilities and my weaknesses to be bare before those closest to me. Relationships are the mirror in which we can see ourselves: the good, the bad and the ugly. We can either be transformed by the constant feedback and continue to open up to key relationships or we can learn to protect and socially isolate to avoid the pain and reality of the mess that we are.

Just as vividly as I remember the broken-hearted moments that I experienced in the past with Joe, I'm sure that you can remember the times of your deepest pain. Interestingly enough, there is a disease correlated to the emotional pain from a broken heart called takotsubo cardiomyopathy. Doctors simply call it broken-heart syndrome as heart complications can arise from the emotional pain of a broken heart.

In fact, in 2016, a woman was airlifted to a Houston hospital with a case of broken-heart syndrome.[1] The doctors thought that she was having a heart attack, but when they looked at her arteries, they were completely clear. The woman, Joanie, shared that she tended to "take things more to heart than other people" and had recently experienced several losses. This was the first documented case of broken-heart syndrome.

According to research at Cleveland Clinic in Ohio, broken-heart syndrome has increased 4-fold since the pandemic of the coronavirus in 2020.[2] Symptoms of broken-heart syndrome can mimic symptoms of a heart attack and include chest pain, shortness of breath, an elevated electrocardiogram and elevated cardiac enzyme levels.[3] Other symptoms can include irregular heartbeat, low blood pressure and even fainting. All the symptoms mimic a heart attack, except when doctors look at the arteries, they are completely clear.

This broken-heart syndrome occurs most exclusively to women after the stress of the loss of a loved one or another emotional event. Doctors believe that a person's reaction emotionally to a stressful event can reduce the heart's ability to pump. A study in New England Journal of Medicine, found that a flood of stress hormones could stun the heart and produce heart spasms that can mimic a heart attack.[4]

Thankfully, I was not airlifted to the hospital because of broken-heart syndrome and I survived my broken heart through the support of friends and family, prayer and meditation and going through the normal stages of grieving. Sometimes, people with cancer suffer from a broken heart and live with unresolved trauma or loss. Dealing with trauma, releasing grief and healing emotionally are all significant aspects to healing physically from cancer.

I remember a conversation with one of my clients with Stage IV lung cancer regarding trauma and grieving. She recounted several painful times in her life where she felt betrayed by people close to her. She lamented, "When my children were young, our church became divided about several theological issues. The topics became heavily debated. Many of us sought to rectify and unify the church body. Others, however, planned a church divide and half the church left. Our church suffered a lot, and I personally struggled as I was trying to glue back the pieces of a broken congregation to no avail. All of my efforts did nothing to effect change or healing. I was numb and unable to process my emotions for many months. A similar situation happened years later with my children's primary school. The community wanted to keep the school private, but many members wanted the school to become public, adopting public school curriculum. We felt strongly as a family that we wanted the school to maintain its private status, and keep the current curriculum the same. The board voted for the school to become public, and I was devastated. I spent many hours trying to voice my opinion, but my words fell on deaf ears. Years later, I feel so much grief bottled up inside of me as a result of these unresolved traumas."

We spent some time that day redesigning the memories that she had of those painful events. My client was able to express emotions that she had forgotten about over the years. I asked her, "What would you say to yourself in those situations, all these years later knowing what you know now about the outcome of your family?"

My client sighed saying, "I would tell myself, you did your best. Your love and concern for your children was your motivation and this was right. In the end, the school changed and your church changed. It wasn't what you wanted. But in the end, your kids turned out all right and you still have your church all these years later. The decisions that others made in those situations were out of your hands."

"Now, how does that feel?" I said after a pause.

My client took a breath in, "It feels better, more serene."

"Let's try something. Now, I want you to try to forgive the people who hurt you in the church split and the decision about your children's school. Go back into the memory, look at each person you need to forgive and tell them that you forgive them." My client paused, closed her eyes and said, "Tom, I forgive you, Sally, I forgive you. I forgive myself. I forgive…."

In the end, my client was able to release those pent-up emotions of grief and move forward with living. Her body responded in an amazing way, and her oncologist told her a couple of months later that the scan of her lungs showed only scar tissue, no tumor was present any longer.

In 2011, a study was released from The National Institute of Mental Health and The National Institute on Drug Abuse on the similarities between emotional and physical pain. Researchers compared the brain scans on an fMRI of individuals who experienced a recent break up compared to what areas of the brain activate after physical pain. Subjects were shown a photograph of their ex-partner and asked to think about the recent break up while their brains were scanned. The scans showed that the same areas in the brain that become active during physical pain, the secondary somatosensory cortex and the dorsal posterior insula, became active after social rejection as well.[5] According to over 500 studies, it doesn't seem to matter if you experience physical pain from a car accident or the emotional pain of going through a divorce, your brain doesn't discern the difference between the two events. To your brain, physical pain and emotional pain are the same.

Some people with cancer struggle to develop authentic relationships with people because they have learned to suppress their emotions after many experiences with rejection and emotional pain. In fact, Lydia Temoshok, a psychologist at UCSF, demonstrated that cancer patients, who kept emotions like anger under the surface or remained ignorant of their existence, had slower recovery rates.[6]

Other cancer patients are simply lonely, and have not figured out how to develop intimate relationships that can bring healing to their broken hearts. Many of us know that poor nutrition, a lack of exercise, obesity and smoking are risk factors to our health. But did you know that loneliness is as big of a risk factor to your health as those factors?

Loneliness has been found to increase your risk of an early death by 20%.[7] Loneliness has been found to affect 1 in 4 people in the U.S. and perhaps this number has increased since the coronavirus pandemic in 2020.

People who reported fewer social connections showed disrupted sleep patterns, altered immune systems, higher levels of inflammation, as well as higher levels of stress hormones. Also, in 28 studies of 180,000 adults, loneliness and social isolation are associated with a 29% increased risk of heart attack and a 32% greater risk of stroke.[8]

As a culture, the Western world is not always the best at prioritizing community over self. Many times, we are so driven and self-focused, that we forget the importance of relational connections.

However, initiating small, micro-connections with people during our day serves to increase the activity of our vagus nerve and to decrease the impact of loneliness.[9] If you see your neighbor outside, go and say hi! If you are going on a walk and you see someone you don't know, introduce yourself and have a conversation with them! Your body will release a powerful drug called oxytocin.

Oxytocin is called the love drug and is released when falling in love, when mothers nurse their babies and even when we interact in small ways with neighbors, grocery store clerks or strangers. Oxytocin helps to create connection, attraction and bonding. This love hormone simply helps to form and deepen relationships. Oxytocin has many health benefits and acts as an anti-stress tonic. Oxytocin counteracts fight or flight stress hormones, acts as an anti-inflammatory agent and triggers the parasympathetic nervous system in order to shift the body into rest, heal and repair mode.[10]

It is important to note that you don't have to breastfeed or fall in love with someone to release oxytocin. In fact, social interactions and building relationships with anyone can increase your body's production of oxytocin. The best way to increase oxytocin is by naturally focusing on ALL social interactions. Oxytocin increases when we learn to "fall in love" over and over again with our spouse, neighbor, family member, friend, co-worker and even through interactions with perfect strangers.[11] Social connections are an essential nutrient and we simply cannot heal without love and connection. Here are some ways to increase your production of oxytocin:

- Physical contact such as hugs, massages, being intimate, shaking hands and breastfeeding
- Essential oils — Studies suggest that certain essential oils like clary sage oil may increase the production of oxytocin
- Making eye contact
- Laughing
- Throwing parties and having friends over for dinner
- Giving and receiving gifts
- Petting a dog, cat or other pet
- Doing "loving kindness" meditation or visualization
- Telling someone you love them
- Listening to calming music
- Speaking to a friend or family member on the phone
- Walking or exercising with someone
- Looking at photos or videos of people you care about[12]

When a cancer patient receives love and support from friends and family, the body increases the production of dopamine, oxytocin, serotonin and endorphins. These hormones have a powerful impact on the body and the immune system.[13] In fact, dopamine, oxytocin, serotonin and endorphins all have been found to decrease inflammation, increase blood circulation, increase oxygen circulation, increase white blood cells, increase red blood cells, increase helper T cells and increase natural killer cells.[14] These are some powerful drugs that are initiated based upon our willingness to engage socially on a day-to-day basis. If you can eat your vegetables for your health, can you also go out of your way to talk to your neighbor, spouse or even your grocery store clerk? If so, you will find immense benefits to your health.

Impressively, breast cancer patients who increased social support reduced their risk of dying by 70%.[15] Further, strong social connections lengthen survival outcomes in those diagnosed with cancer on average by 25%.[16] Thus, building strong social connections is essential to longevity and is part of the healing process for cancer patients.

I still remember a pivotal conversation with my client who had been diagnosed with ovarian cancer regarding her relationships. Pam called me with such excitement and zeal, "It's a miracle! You aren't going to believe what happened this weekend! I had my sister in law, Connie, over for 8 hours and we talked and talked and talked, and I cried through most of it, but we reconciled our relationship. I still can't believe what happened!" I was overjoyed at her miracle. Pam had been disconnected from her family for 20-plus years. Specifically, she hadn't spoken to her sister-in-law and her niece for about 20 years. At a wedding, her niece had said something to her that was very rude, and she couldn't let it go. When she had done a shower for her sister-in-law's daughter, Pam did all of the work and no one offered to help her with cleaning afterwards. She described how her feet were swollen and her blood sugars had plummeted, but she kept on working. She felt very offended that no one offered to help her, especially her sister-in-law, Connie. She cut the relationships off as a result (there had been other moments in their relationships where Pam had been offended and over time, the issues were never resolved).

A few weeks prior to this conversation, I had been in a session with my client, Pam, and I felt like we needed a breakthrough. Pam still had not told any of her family members that she had cancer despite the fact that she had been doing treatments for over a year. There was something that needed to be addressed and forgiveness was just not happening. I said the following to Pam in our session: "Pam, I just get the sense that you are struggling to forgive family members because you are offended at what they have done in the past. Let me try to explain offense to you and see if it makes sense to you. Offense is an internal process that happens when we look at what a person says and does and we judge them and feel strongly that they should have said it this way or done it that way. And surely if they cared about us at all, they would have noticed and helped us or done it differently. Offense is an internal process that happens when we act in pride, self-righteousness and judge another person's motives and intent without seeking understanding. Do you think that you have done this in past relationships with family members?" I shared my thoughts about offense as I had found several times I had clients with cancer struggle to forgive because offense blocked them from doing so.

Pam listened intently and decided to buy a CD series on the topic of "offense" to listen to while she drove to North Carolina with her husband. I couldn't believe my ears when she told me about her experience learning about offense. Pam told me the following when she got home from her trip to North Carolina, "I listened to the CDs on offense the whole way there and the whole way back. I cried for an entire week because I said to myself, 'I thought that it was their fault for what happened and why we were no longer in relationship with one another. But, if I was the one who was wrong because I took offense, I didn't think that I could bear that truth.' But it was true in the end. I was wrong because I didn't process everything in a healthy way and I got offended. I am ready to release my offenses and tell them about my cancer diagnosis." Shortly after she got home from North Carolina, Pam set up meetings with her sister-in-law and her niece. She opened up about her diagnosis and about her past hurts. She was finally able to hear their perspectives on what happened and forgive fully.

I still remember how powerful of a miracle the forgiveness and reconciliation was for Pam when she said the following to me months later, "I am alienated by no one in my life, I feel love from everyone. This is the first time that I have felt like this in my life."

As we will explore further in this section on relationships, it is not just any type of social connection or community that makes the difference. It is the quality and type of relational connection that makes a difference in our healing process. Many people with cancer have relationships that need to be reconciled like my client Pam and others have to learn to dig deeper in their relationships. It's one thing to have a lot of friends and it's another thing to have 2-3 friends with whom you can share anything. The first step in Section 1 is about finding self-awareness and emotional expression to the point where you can express yourself in an authentic way. The next step is finding your people, the ones with whom you are able to be vulnerable and express yourself: the good, the bad and the ugly, and find affirmation and love instead of shame and rejection.

Section 2: Relationships Reflect Me: What Do You See?

Chapter 2: My Soul Deserves Peace

Eagerly awaiting the performance, I glanced across the room and noticed someone sitting alone near the front row. A strange compulsion to go and sit next to the lone stranger came over my entire body. Taken aback, I dismissed the bizarre compulsion and stayed glued to my seat. What was that about? I thought to myself. I had never felt an odd inclination to go and sit next to a perfect stranger before and I wasn't about to test my intuition.

A few minutes later, the mysterious stranger was called up to the stage to perform an original song. Mesmerized by his song, I found myself drawn into his energy to the point where my earlier inclination didn't seem so insane. Okay, I thought to myself, at least I will find him afterwards and meet him. I wondered if the unexpected connection that I felt would mean anything.

At the end of the evening, I started to make my way over to the stranger. I felt anxious, yet determined to follow through. Hesitating, I decided to take off my boots as they made me quite tall and I didn't want to make an overbearing impression. Also, it seemed like the mysterious performer was quite short compared to me.

Trying to act casual, like I wasn't calculating my every move, I slowly walked over to engage with my target. I stuck out my hand to introduce myself and heard the following words tumble out of my mouth without the intention of ever speaking them: "Hi! My name is Megan, are you from Latin America?" Embarrassed at my forthright introduction and my brash assumption of his potential ethnic background, I realized that I was scoping him out as a potential mate. After breaking up with Joe and pouring my guts out to my friend Sjhira, I had my heart set on marrying someone from the Latina culture.

"I'm Eugene and I'm from the tip of Africa. South Africa, not Latin America, but I get that a lot." He flashed a magnanimous grin that made me feel more at ease. At least he couldn't read my thoughts. His accent was endearing and I was very intrigued by his energy. We chatted for another few minutes before he awkwardly said, "One time, I had the opportunity to talk to a beautiful girl or to help tear down the set after a performance. I chose to tear down the set." And with that, he was gone.

What a strange night, I thought, as I walked to the parking lot. Apparently, we had mutual friends and we had simply not been introduced yet. It was possible that I would run into him again.

Fast forward to Christmas, I had traveled home for the holidays and was enjoying some time off of work. Somehow, Eugene had gotten my phone number and reached out one night to talk. After the first night that I met him, we ran into each other a few more times at birthday parties and other events. He somehow managed to get my phone number before I left for the holidays.

Feeling nervous, I answered his phone call and chatted to him about nothing and everything all at the same time. Hours later, I looked at my phone and realized that it was 3:00 am! I couldn't believe it. We had been talking for 4 hours! I had never spoken on the phone with anyone that long. From that first night onward, we would speak until early in the morning for a few weeks prior to having a "define the relationship" conversation. I remember it going something like this: "So do you want to see where this goes? I have to tell you that my visa is going to expire and I may have to move back to Cape Town, South Africa." Eugene explained with a question in his eyes.

"I can travel." I answered with enthusiasm and abandon.

Nothing like my first relationship, my connection with Eugene was very different than anything I had ever experienced. In my relationship with Joe, we were so similar that people would often mistake us for brother and sister. However, Eugene and I were the classic opposites attract couple. Eugene's outgoing, witty and magnanimous personality intrigued me. I was more introverted, emotional and calculated in a relationship. I was amazed at how easy it was for Eugene to perform his music in public settings and how easily he would connect with people. Everywhere he went, Eugene would meet people and make new friends.

We started dating after the 1st of the year in 2009 and started spending every free moment together. He loved to cook and would often make meals for the two of us. He also loved to make music and would often share his new songs with me. When we first started dating, I didn't seem to need to sleep. We would talk for over 4 hours a night. Then, I would sleep for 4-5 hours and wake up full of energy! I was shocked at how healthy I felt despite how little I slept and how little food I ate. I was living on love.

I walked around with a cheesy smile on my face, remembering bits and pieces of our conversation from the night before. I felt like everything was right with the world and my mind was completely consumed with thinking about Eugene and every facet of our relationship.

Maybe you remember this feeling as well? The euphoria of love literally comes from love chemicals being released in your body including: dopamine, testosterone, estrogen, vasopressin and oxytocin. Love is the best medicine. Our body releases chemicals based upon receiving and expressing love. Interactions of bonding and connection that are infused with love can change your biochemistry. Any positive change in your biochemistry will impact your health trajectory over time, if positive social interactions are sustained.

What controls the release of love medicine in the body? Your vagus nerve does. The vagus nerve is part of your parasympathetic nervous system and connects your 3 brains: your gut, heart and brain. Current research points to the fact that our body relies upon input, information and even decision making from the gut, heart and the brain; instead of just from the brain as previously thought! Your heart has over 40,000 neurons and a network of neurotransmitters. The heart has been found to feel, think and decide for itself while communicating to the brain through the vagus nerve. Your gut has over 100 million neurons and is responsible for producing 95% of serotonin in the body.[1] Some signals or communication begin in the gut or the heart and flow up to the brain and other signals begin in the brain and flow downwards through the vagus nerve to the heart and the gut.[2]

Anil Rayvanshi writes, "Recent studies have shown that the heart sends signals to the brain that are not only understood by it but also obeyed. Scientists have discovered neural pathways and mechanisms whereby input from the heart to the brain inhibits or facilitates the brain's electrical activity – just like what the gut is capable of doing. Thus, both the gut and the heart help in the overall thought process."[3]

The vagus nerve passes messages between the mind and the body millions of times over the course of a day. Vagus is Latin for wandering and the vagus nerve quite literally wanders throughout the body, exiting the brain stem at the base of the skull. If you press your fingers deep into your neck on the pulse point, you are close to your vagus nerve.

How do you activate your vagus nerve? Your vagus nerve is like a muscle, the more you use it, the stronger it becomes. You can activate your vagus nerve by deep, abdominal breathing which allows your body to relax and activate the parasympathetic nervous system. Connecting with a friend, spouse, neighbor or even a stranger can stimulate the vagus nerve. Our vagal tone is also reflected in our ability to rapidly activate the parasympathetic nervous system. Thus, practices that activate the parasympathetic nervous system can influence your vagal tone, including, coffee enemas, meditation, sensory-depravation tanks (floating) and PEMF.[4] Studies have found that PEMF can increase heart rate variability and increase vagus stimulation.[5] Further, studies have found that higher vagal tone is associated with greater closeness to others and more altruistic behavior.[6]

In the Loving-kindness Meditation Study on vagal tone, participants went through a 6-week course training them how to cultivate love, compassion and goodwill towards themselves and others.[7] Meditation and social interactions were recorded throughout the course. Fredrickson tested the participants' vagal tone before and after the study. In the study, participants were instructed to sit and think compassionately about others by silently repeating phrases like "May you feel safe, may you feel happy, may you feel healthy and may you live with ease." Participants were further instructed to keep returning to these thoughts whenever their minds wandered.

Compared to the control group, the participants who meditated experienced an overall increase in positive emotions after the 6-week course including: joy, interest, amusement, serenity and hope. Further, the emotional and psychological changes correlated with a greater sense of connectedness to others. The study also showed an improvement in both vagal tone and heart rate variability compared to the control group, who did not participate in the 6-week course.

Meditation without an increase in social interactions did not result in a more toned vagus nerve. At the end of the study, meditators who increased their number of social interactions on a daily basis felt more socially connected, became happier and experienced improvement in their vagal tone. For those who meditated at the same rate as other participants, but did not report feeling any closer to others or any change in how many social interactions they experienced on a daily basis, there was also no change in the tone of their vagus nerve.

If making relational connections are so valuable and important to our mental, emotional and physical health, why don't we all prioritize relationships? One reason is that we have all experienced emotional pain, rejection and loss and some of us have unresolved emotional pain. If you watch a toddler interacting with people, they are open, excited to connect and don't easily withdraw from people. However, if you watch an adult in social interactions, you can almost see the walls of protection around their hearts because of past rejection, betrayal or conflict. How do we reverse the effects of emotional pain in relationships? One way to discover peace and openness to new relationships is the practice of forgiveness.

Forgiveness is a letting go and surrendering process that many people avoid due to the fear of being hurt again and due to a lack of understanding of the process of forgiveness. On the other hand, some people use un-forgiveness as a shield to protect themselves from being hurt again. Unfortunately, if we harbor un-forgiveness and bitterness within one relationship, our heart becomes hardened and we bring mistrust into other relationships. All of our relationships begin to be distorted and under siege. Further, emotions released in the body, as a result of bitterness, cause a reaction in our stress response system that changes our biochemistry and breaks down our metabolic reserves.[8]

I remember vividly the day that my client with col-rectal cancer sat staring straight ahead, saying to me, "I know that I need to forgive my mom, but I don't know how. I feel stuck." I empathized with my client that forgiveness is not always easy. Over the process of many sessions, my client had revealed deep pain in her relationship with her mother. As a child, my client Lisa had felt emotionally abandoned, neglected and even verbally assaulted by her mother. She felt that her mother was a narcissist, and that every conversation was about her and never about Lisa. The emotional pain was so intense and all encompassing that Lisa struggled to figure out how to move beyond her raw emotions to forgive the person who had hurt her more than anyone else in her life. Grappling with her decision whether to forgive or not, Lisa reasoned, "I mean, shouldn't someone be held accountable for the pain that they have caused?"

"Let's do an exercise together and ask the spiritual realm for help in the process of forgiving your mom." I heard myself saying that out loud at the same time that I realized the right strategy for Lisa. I asked Lisa to lie down on the couch as her husband said, "I'm going to leave and give you two some space." I placed a hand on Lisa's shoulder and asked for divine intervention, "Lisa is struggling to forgive her mom right now. Can you empower her to forgive her mom?" Then I paused, holding my breath and waiting for the answer in eager anticipation.

All of a sudden, I witnessed Lisa exhale loudly as tears poured down her face. Sitting up from her position, she continued to inhale and exhale loudly while tears streamed uncontrollably. A look of surprise and deep contemplation broke only when Lisa realized that I was waiting for insight into what had occurred, "I saw an image of Jesus on the cross. He said to me, 'Forgive them, for they know not what they do.' I grew up Catholic, but I never spent much time thinking about the cross. In fact, I found it to be violent and terrifying. As I watched Jesus on the cross forgive those who murdered Him, I was overcome with compassion for my mom. I forgive my mom. I can forgive my mom. Wow. It's done."

Being one of the most profound experiences that I have ever had with a client, I will never forget this moment with Lisa. After that day, she noticed a profound shift in her relationship with her mom. She was no longer consumed with anger and thoughts of resentment towards what her mom had done and not done for her. In fact, when her mom called, she wasn't as bothered by her narcissistic tendencies. The image that empowered Lisa to forgive was the moment of freedom that she had been searching for her entire adult life.

When we have unresolved trauma and relational conflict in our lives, we tend to live in a sympathetic dominant fight or flight state, which causes difficulty in creating relational connections. In fact, we can transition to a neuropeptide state. Neuroception is how the brain processes in order to determine whether a person or situation is safe or dangerous. Researchers have discovered that people can go into a neurocepid state, which means that people can lose the capacity to make social connections. For example, trauma victims in a constant state of fight or flight move into a fight-flight-freeze mode with the nervous system hyper vigilant on detecting a predator while unable to focus on making social connections.[9]

How does someone who experienced trauma transition from a neurocepid state of being unable to make social connections into a state of parasympathetic dominance where their nervous system doesn't view everyone as a threat? Forgiveness and releasing offense are two keys to moving out of a neurocepid state.

Forgiveness has been associated with lowered blood pressure, lowered risk of heart attack and a stronger immune system. However, un-forgiveness has been found to dampen the immune system and make it worse at fighting off viruses and bacteria. In fact, negative emotions from un-forgiveness trigger a cascade of chemicals and hormones that impede the immune system's response in the body. On the other hand, forgiveness halts patterns of stress in the body and works to rebalance stress hormones, which can improve an immune system's response.[10] No wonder why cancer patients experience such a dramatic shift in their physical body after forgiving people who have hurt them in the past.

Do you want to take a step closer towards healing? Start by choosing to forgive and find yourself freed from the stress of holding onto bitterness.

The 5 Keys to Forgiveness:

1. Forgiveness is a choice. You will never feel like forgiving someone. You can use your will as a weapon and choose forgiveness despite how you feel and your feelings will shift as a result. "Today, I decided to forgive you. Not because you apologized or because you acknowledged the pain that you caused me, but because my soul deserves peace." ~Najwa Zebian

2. Sometimes, you need to forgive multiple times, even daily until you are completely free from bitterness.

3. Forgiveness sometimes means reconciliation with the person who hurt you, but not always. Sometimes, reconciliation is not possible, but forgiveness is necessary for your own health and ability to have new, positive relationships.

4. Taking offense in relational situations can hinder our ability to forgive. What is offense? When someone behaves in a certain way, our tendency can be to make a snap judgment on why they did or said something. We can easily become offended with what someone says or does if we do not seek to understand their thoughts and motives behind the statement or behavior. Many times, my clients with cancer are trapped in bitterness because of offense. We can choose to release past offenses and this will help break a pattern of taking offense in relational interactions. The next time someone does something that you don't understand, seek to understand why he or she did what he or she did and you will stop the trap of offense.

For example, my client with ovarian cancer, Pam, became offended at her sister-in-law after she hosted her daughter's wedding shower. During and after the shower, Pam was feeling the weight of responsibility in hosting the event and was feeling not well because of her symptoms of Type I Diabetes. She noticed her feet swelling up as she gathered plates to wash in the kitchen. No one offered to help her clean. Internally, she became increasingly mad and offended that she was left alone to host and clean up after the party. After the event, she was so embittered and offended by the lack of help from her sister-in-law that she cut off the relationship entirely.

It wasn't until 20-years later that Pam realized she had been part of the problem because she took offense without asking for help or even explaining to her sister-in-law how she had been feeling that day. It is so common for us to assume what someone is thinking and feeling and to make a snap judgment against them. This offense breaks relationships and causes bitterness to solidify. Do you have a pattern of taking offense to what people in your life say and do or what they don't say or do?

5. Un-forgiveness can lead to hatred, malice and even retaliation. Our inability to forgive one person in our life can lead to an inability to trust and open our hearts to new relationships that come our way. Forgive so that you can also move forward into healthy patterns of relating in new relationships.

Agnes Sanford stated the following, "As we practice the work of forgiveness, we discover more and more that forgiveness and healing are one."

A client with Stage 4-lung cancer went into spontaneous remission after discovering her internal relational habit of taking offense. She realized that from a young age, she compared how she was treated with her stepsiblings, and always felt like she got the short end of the stick. Because of this, she learned a life-long habit of judging people's motives and taking offense in relational interactions. Every major trauma in her life had a common theme: there was an injustice and that injustice targeted her in a personal way. She would become offended as a result. She kept many people at a distance and wasn't very open and trusting in relationships. She was skeptical and cynical at best.

Once she began to notice her habit of taking offense and started to change her way of internally processing relational interactions, her emotions shifted in a profound way. Her relationships improved rapidly and she began to be more open with her family and friends. After 6 months of digging deep into her emotional, spiritual and relational root issues, her oncologist found no tumor mass in her lungs, only scar tissue where the tumor previously resided. The body is truly wired for spontaneous remission! Now, find your companion workbook to do the exercises involved with forgiveness and releasing offense.

Section 2: Relationships Reflect Me: What Do You See?

Chapter 3: Into Me You See

Sitting in Starbucks, I can still feel the twinge in my heart today as I remember how the tears streamed down my face after my date with Joe. It's happening again. Somehow, I find myself in Starbucks, crying, this time for something I have yet to understand fully.

Why is it that I leave every date crying at the end? I ask internally. It had been a few weeks now that I found myself crying after every single date with Joe. Confused and bewildered, I say abruptly, "Let's get out of here." Without a word or hesitation, Joe stood up and took me home.

Our new and exciting relationship took a sharp turn after 3-months of bliss. I couldn't quite pinpoint what was wrong. However, without fail, at the end of every date, tears would stream down my face spontaneously. Emotionally, I couldn't reach him anymore. We had been emotionally in sync for so long. Now, it felt like I kept hitting a brick wall of Joe's pain, bitterness and anger towards his dad. It just sat there and grew like mold, shutting me out of the deep, safe place that I had learned to depend so heavily upon.

A couple of weeks after that day in Starbucks, I found myself skiing in Colorado with my family. My mom and I got massages one day and as I was relaxing, I heard a voice say, "If you break up with him, I will heal him." In shock, I froze internally at the weight of the words. After waiting for nearly 6 years to date my first love, I was to break up with him? It seemed absolutely insane at first.

However, after reflecting upon the words that I had clearly heard, I knew that I could not keep Joe hostage to a relationship that was never going to be enough to bring healing to the deeper wounds that he had sustained from his dad. Breaking up soon after this period of time, I didn't fully understand the psychological warfare that destroyed our intimate bond. Only after time, I began to understand more what had occurred between us. We all can experience defensive reactions to feeling vulnerable depending upon the types of attachments we developed with our main caregivers as children. We can learn to defend against feeling vulnerable by seeking isolation, withdrawing or becoming inaccessible.

Joe's ability to give and receive love became impaired at the end of our relationship because of the bitterness he was feeling towards his father. In essence, Joe sabotaged our intimate relationship without conscious awareness because he couldn't resolve his embittered emotions towards his father.

When we don't believe that we are worth being loved in a certain way, we can sabotage the best relationship of our life. When we are struggling to resolve inner turmoil, we may unintentionally sabotage our closest relationships. Vulnerability and the ability to have deep intimacy in relationships are both qualities that require introspection and growth in emotional intelligence. It requires us resolving past emotional trauma, betrayal and rejection so that we can trust and build healthy bonds.

Thus, my relationship with myself is contingent upon my relationships with others, and my relationships with others are contingent upon my relationship with myself. So, what comes first, the chicken or the egg? In other words, do I address my relationship with others or my relationship with myself first? It doesn't' matter where you begin, as long as you begin. They will both influence each other. We are uniquely complicated beings, and it can take some unraveling to find the essence of who we are and why we struggle to express ourselves in an authentic manner. Introspection is to self-awareness as vulnerability is to building intimate relationships.

If I am unaware of my emotions, thought patterns and beliefs, I will struggle to open up to another human being. **The word intimacy literally translates to "into me you see."** How can someone see into me if I cannot see into me?

Vulnerability becomes nearly impossible when we have learned to protect ourselves from being hurt by hiding emotions from others and from ourselves.

Many of us have not learned to trust others enough to open up raw and deep emotions. Often, children make inner decisions to change how they relate to others because of an emotional wound. I had this experience as a child, but didn't realize that I had made an internal decision until I was conflicted by my inability to show vulnerability towards women. In order to find my natural ability to open up to women again, I had to first discover what happened during childhood that hindered me. Once I was able to connect to the memory that held the maladaptive core belief, "I cannot trust women with deep emotions," I redesigned the memory by forgiving and making a new decision to trust women with my emotions again.

We all develop psychological defenses on the subconscious level in early childhood. When a child experiences deprivation, rejection or the fear of separation, he or she can develop psychological defenses and even unhealthy attachments with a caregiver that can set the stage for unhealthy relational attachments for the rest of their life.

In childhood, the psychological defenses serve to reduce a child's experience of emotional pain, anxiety, sadness, shame and other overwhelming feelings. In a situation of life-threatening trauma, psychological defenses protect a child.[1] The development of an infant's mind is completely dependent on people in their immediate environment for the first 2 years of his or her life.[2] It is nearly impossible for all of the infant's needs to be met even in a good family environment. Thus, children adapt in order to survive and may develop unhealthy attachment patterns or psychological defenses that will manifest in adult relationships.

The development of a healthy, secure attachment between an infant and a primary caregiver determines how well the child transitions to being a healthy, functioning adult. Children become attached to whoever functions as their primary caregiver, and whether or not that attachment is secure or insecure will impact the rest of their lives. A secure attachment develops best in a relationship that is both in sync and emotionally attuned. Attunement is the sense that a child feels understood and that their primary caregiver is meeting their emotional needs. When infants and caregivers are in sync on an emotional level, they also become in sync on a physical level.[3] Further, when children have a secure attachment with their primary caregiver, they easily become in sync with their environment and the people around them to develop self-awareness, empathy, impulse control and self-motivation.

Babies cannot regulate their own emotional states. They rely on their caregiver to help regulate emotions. When their primary caregiver shares love and connection, the infant maintains a steady heartbeat with a low level of stress hormones, but when the emotional state of the caretaker is disrupted, the physiology of the infant changes as a result. An attachment researcher from Edinburgh, Colwyn Trevarthen found that infants learn musically from their mother's voice starting in the womb. Further, she discovered that an infant coordinates rhythmic body movements to act in sync with the mind of their primary caregiver.[4]

There are 4 main childhood attachment patterns that have been discovered in attachment research: secure, avoidant, anxious and disorganized.[5] The secure child grows up with a parent who is sensitive and responsive during interactions. The parent is attuned and available to the child, and the child feels safe and seen in a secure attachment. When the child is hurting, the parent responds with compassion. A child with a secure attachment to a parent is well adjusted with fewer defenses in relationships as an adult. Securely attached infants act distressed when their parent leaves and delighted when they return. After a check-in for reassurance, securely attached infants can settle in and resume play after their primary caregiver leaves. Infants in secure relationships learn to communicate their frustrations, distress, interests, preferences, goals and their emerging selves.

A secure attachment in childhood promotes self-reliance, empathy and the ability to help others who are in a state of distress. Researchers have found that securely attached children build an internal locus of control, which is a key factor for healthy coping throughout life.[6] Securely attached children easily learn what makes them feel good and what makes them and others feel bad. They also learn what situations they can control and when they need help. This sets the stage for children to play an active role as an adult when faced with difficult situations.

The best type of attachment that promotes healthy relationships and healthy coping skills in adulthood is the secure attachment. Many children grow up in homes where they do not develop a secure attachment with a primary caregiver. Children with histories of abuse and neglect learn that their emotions, fear and crying do not register with their caregiver. Thus, nothing they do or say will bring attention or help. Unfortunately, this will condition a child to give up when they face challenges as an adult.

Further, when a primary caregiver cannot tune into their baby's reality and meet the baby's physical and emotional needs, the baby adapts to meet the expectations of their caregiver. The baby will perceive that something is wrong with them and shame will permeate the worldview of the child. Negative, maladaptive beliefs will undergird the perception of the child, leading to self-destructive behaviors and a poor ability to cope with life's stressors in adulthood. In addition, negative self-perceptions from childhood can set the stage for people to be traumatized as adults. When the type of attachment does not allow for internal security or causes the child to conclude that they are a terrible person, this sets the stage for unhealthy relational attachments in adulthood along with an inability to handle life's demands.[7]

The second attachment type is the avoidant attachment pattern. This attachment can develop when a parent is unavailable and emotionally distant to their child. The adult may be preoccupied with their own life, unaware of the child, oblivious or insensitive to their needs. When the child is hurting, the adult has no response. Often in the avoidant attachment, the parent discourages the child from crying. The child who develops avoidant attachment patterns learns to be self-sufficient at an early age and learns to want little from others with minimal interactions. Children who have an avoidant attachment pattern have been found to have chronically increased heart rates with consistent hyper arousal in their stress response systems. Many times, children with an avoidant attachment pattern do not cry when their primary caregiver leaves and they choose to ignore the parent when they come back. It has been noted by researchers that parents who develop avoidant attachment patterns with their children struggle to hold and snuggle with their babies and don't use facial expressions to interact with them.

The third type of attachment is the anxious attachment pattern. This type of attachment develops when a parent is inconsistent and contradictory in their behavior. At times, this parent is responsive, but other times, the parent is emotionally unavailable. The child becomes confused and insecure. The child never knows what type of response they will receive from their caregiver. In this attachment, the child can become clingy and act desperate towards their parent. The child can also become distrustful and insecure. This defensive reaction causes the child to cling to the parent in order to have their needs met. When a caregiver attempts to leave a child with an anxious attachment pattern, this child draws attention to themselves by crying and yelling while staying focused on their parent instead of playing.[8]

The last form of attachment is the disorganized attachment pattern. This pattern develops for many potential reasons: lack of financial stability; PTSD or trauma that is unresolved for the primary caregiver; physical or emotional abuse; or the recent death of a loved one. Sometimes, the disorganized attachment pattern develops when the parent is physically or emotionally abusive to their child. The child can psychologically detach, moving out of their body to avoid the trauma. The child becomes torn from wanting and fearing their caregiver, and the child becomes emotionally disconnected.[9] Infants are unable to figure out how to engage with caregivers because their caregivers are both the source of distress and comfort. In the disorganized pattern of attachment, infants will look at their parent and then quickly turn away. The infant is unable to choose between drawing close to their caregiver and avoiding their caregiver, as **they don't know to whom they belong.**

Abused children are overly sensitive to the slightest expression of anger. They become easily scared and defensive. Throughout their childhood, they overreact to peers' anger and aggression, don't discern the needs of their peers and easily lose control of their impulses. Unfortunately, as a result, these children experience a lot of rejection from their peers. Abused children spend more time alone, watching TV or playing video games.[10]

Besides physical and emotional abuse, financial stress can cause such instability in a family that the primary caregiver attaches in a disorganized manner to their child.[11] Further, a primary caregiver that is preoccupied with their own trauma such as the recent death of a loved one may be too emotionally unstable to offer comfort and protection to their infant. For example, pregnant women who were in the World Trade Center in 2001 during terrorist attacks were found to have an increased vulnerability to developing a disorganized attachment with their infant because of this traumatic experience.[12] Further, holocaust survivors, victims of assault or rape were also found to have a risk of developing a disorganized attachment with their children.

Another study on 9/11 discovered that children whose mothers were diagnosed with PTSD or depression after the terrorist attack had a 6-fold increased risk of developing significant emotional problems and a 11-fold increased risk of becoming hyper-aggressive.[13] Another study on PTSD found that the reactions of children to painful events were by in large determined by how calm or stressed their parents appeared to be.[14] When children were hospitalized with severe burns, if they had a secure attachment with their mother, they needed less morphine than those children who did not feel safe with their mothers.

By Kindergarten, children with a disorganized attachment pattern with their primary caregiver demonstrated behaviors of aggression, disengagement and showed physiological signs of stress: increased heart rate, heart rate variability issues and decreased immune factors.[15] Further, children with a disorganized attachment pattern were found to have a higher risk of developing psychiatric problems.

Karlen Lyons-Ruth performed an extensive study on the disorganized attachment by video-taping a child's interaction with their primary caregiver at 6-months, 12-months, 18-months, 5-years and 7-8 years with a follow up when the child became an adult at 20-years of age.[16] Lyons-Ruth engaged her research with high-risk families. All of the families were considered to be in poverty and half of the moms were single moms. Lyons-Ruth discovered that the moms were too preoccupied with their own issues to care for their infants. Some of the moms interacted with their children in intrusive and hostile manners. Other moms showed signs of helplessness and fear, not greeting their children when they came back into the room, not picking up their children when they were distressed and not attuning with their child's emotions and needs. The moms in the study had histories of physical abuse, domestic violence, sexual abuse and parental loss.[17]

When the children with disorganized attachment patterns were followed-up at 20-years of age, most were found to be unstable with many impulsive behaviors including: excessive spending, promiscuous sex, substance abuse, reckless driving, binge eating, anger and suicidal behavior. Lyons-Ruth found that children who experienced extreme maternal disengagement and poor attunement during the first 2 years of their life developed symptoms of dissociation as young adults.

Attachment patterns with a primary caregiver in childhood can have a huge impact on relational connections and coping skills in adulthood. Children who don't feel safe in infancy have trouble regulating moods and emotional responses as adults. Further, a lack of safety in a primary caregiving relationship leads to an impaired sense of inner reality and excessive clinging to self-damaging behavior. The quality of early caregiving appears to be critical to preventing mental health problems independent of other traumas.[18]

A comprehensive study of attachment patterns in 2,000 infants in normal middle-class environments found that 62% developed secure attachments, 15% developed avoidant attachments, 9% developed anxious attachments and 15% developed disorganized attachments.[19] This study showed that the child's gender and basic temperament have negligible correlation with the development of attachment patterns. In fact, children with difficult temperaments were not more likely to develop a disorganized attachment style.

This suggests that treatment not only needs to address traumatic events but also the consequences of not having been mirrored, attuned to properly or given consistent care and affection by a primary caregiver. The goal of relational health is to be able to restore the ability to sync with close relationships. Being in sync with oneself and others requires integration of body-based senses: vision, hearing, touch and balance. Being in sync with an infant looks like sharing funny faces, giving hugs and expressing delight or disapproval at the right moments. Restoring the ability to sync with others takes a comprehensive approach of both internal and relational attunement. Some therapies that can help this process include: joining a choir or band, joining chamber music, dancing in rhythm and reciprocity, getting a massage and exercising self-awareness through journaling and meditation.[20] We will share more of these strategies in Section 3 during our exploration of trauma.

Finally, let's briefly explore the 4 attachment patterns in romantic relationships to understand how our attachments to a primary caregiver can affect our relationships as adults. There are 4 different attachment styles in romantic relationships: secure, dismissive-avoidant, anxious-preoccupied and fearful-avoidant.[21] In a secure attachment, both parties can be honest, open and equal. Both partners are independent, yet loving with no drama. There will be less psychological defenses against intimacy and love in a relationship where both parties can securely attach.

In the dismissive-avoidant attachment pattern, a person would seek isolation, feel pseudo-independent and primarily focus on self-sufficiency within the context of their romantic relationship. A person who operates in the dismissive-avoidant pattern would not be able to acknowledge their own needs or the needs of others. They would quite literally dismiss or disregard their partner's needs and emotionally distance themselves from their partner, detaching and denying the importance of the relationship.

A person who is insecure, unsure of their partner's feelings and unsafe in close relationships may be operating out of an anxious-preoccupied attachment pattern. They may become clingy, demanding or possessive. In this attachment style, the person seeks to have their partner rescue them or complete them.

The last pattern is the fearful-avoidant attachment style. In this pattern, the partner will manifest an ambivalent state, demonstrating fear when their partner comes too close and fear when their partner becomes too distant. The person operating from this attachment pattern can become trapped in a defensive reaction to love where they move close to love someone, but when they become too close, they pull back because of fear that they will be hurt. The partner who operates in the fearful-avoidant pattern will be clingy at times and yet will feel trapped when the other person draws too close. Thus, the other person in the relationship will feel confused by the unpredictable nature of the relationship while the fearful-avoidant partner will become moody, suppressing emotions at the same time that they feel overwhelmed by emotions.

Our attachment style as an adult will many times be created from the attachment pattern and psychological defenses that we developed throughout childhood as we related to our primary caregiver. We can begin to notice these patterns when we reflect on our upbringing and how we relate to our romantic partners. We may begin to tune in and hear a critical thought pattern that comes against our truest sense of self. This inner voice interferes with self-expression, diminishes our sense of identity and tries to sabotage our relationships. This inner voice stems from maladaptive core beliefs that solidified as we related with our primary caregiver in unhealthy attachment patterns.

The first step to shift our attachment patterns as adults is to examine potential ways that we have learned to protect ourselves from emotional pain. Go to the companion workbook now to answer some reflective questions about your past.

Section 2: Relationships Reflect Me: What Do You See?

Chapter 4: Come Out of Hiding

Standing outside of my dorm room, I struggled to breathe. Something was wrong. I couldn't catch a breath, and my heart felt like it was beating out of my chest. My thoughts were racing; I couldn't follow them and I felt overwhelmed. I grabbed for my phone and called the first person that came to mind, my childhood friend, Becca.

"Hey, Becca, are you there? Hi, how are you? I don't know what's wrong, I can't breathe. My heart is beating super-fast and I can't think straight. Something is wrong. I don't know what it is." My thoughts and emotions tumbled out of me as I began to hyperventilate and share with Becca all of my jumbled thoughts. I quite literally vomited my thoughts and feelings to Becca and in the end, I felt better. It took 45-minutes of me talking and talking and talking, but I finally could catch my breath and my heart slowed down to a normal pattern.

Finally, I could sleep. This would be my first of many panic attacks during my first year of college.

Most nights before bed, I would find a friend with whom I could talk to until my thoughts calmed, my heart slowed down and I felt that I could fall asleep without wrestling with panic the whole night.

I was unaware that I had poor mental health until I found myself in a panic every night. I was struggling to cope with the demands of life. Everything was stressful for me: from picking my major, to deciding when and how to study, to picking an extracurricular activity, to the overall picture of what I wanted to do with my life. The weight of the world was on my shoulders every day. What was I going to do with my one life?

Everything in high school was planned and packaged for me, I would show up and my schedule was packed from sun up to sun down every day. I literally would not have a second to think or unpack my day. It all just caught up to me: the continual running, striving and performing day in and day out to create the perfect resume to be accepted into the perfect college and to live my "dream life." It seemed flawlessly scripted in my mind until I showed up to Vanderbilt University and realized that I had no idea what I was doing and worse yet, I had no idea whom I was. I lived among a sea of people who probably could outperform me on the piano, on the volleyball court, in the classroom and all of a sudden, what made me unique in high school didn't matter anymore. Everyone else at Vanderbilt University was the valedictorian of their high school class and had crafted the perfect resume just like me. So now, who was I?

Good mental health is the balance between life's demands and our potential to face those demands.[1] Sometimes, we lack the coping skills and the internal processing habits to be able to express emotions that hinder us in meeting life's demands. Many of us were not raised in homes where we were taught to openly share our emotions. As adults, we may lack the basic level of emotional intelligence needed to pinpoint what we feel and why. This can become a huge hindrance to good mental health.

So here I am, in college, having panic attacks and needing to unravel all that led me to the place of poor mental health. I felt that I could not cope with the demands of college, partly because I didn't know what I wanted to do with my life, but mainly because I didn't know who I was.

One of the best ways to come out of depression or a panic attack is to admit that you are depressed or in a state of panic. It doesn't matter necessarily how you become aware that you are depressed, just that gain the awareness that you need. You may notice by yourself that you are depressed or someone close to you may point out that you are depressed. I remember after my friend, Sherry, died of breast cancer, I was in a fog. I remember going to the YMCA to swim feeling completely out of body and not myself. It wasn't until I called my mentor on the phone and explained some of the patterns that I was noticing about myself that I gained the clarity needed to move out of a state of depression. My mentor listened to me as I explained, "I feel so unmotivated and dull. I wake up late every day and I have to force myself to go to the YMCA to swim. I feel like I am in a fog. Everything around me feels unreal and I feel spacey and disconnected with reality."

He responded after I shared more details and said, "I think that you may be struggling with depression because of the death of Sherry." As soon as he said those words, it all made sense. The brain fog, confusion, lack of motivation, it was all pointing to depression. I was in one of the stages of grieving. Once I realized this fact, I was able to finish the stages of grieving and accept the reality that Sherry died. When you admit that you are depressed, you can then come out of it.

Learning to understand how we feel and why we feel that way happens best in intimate relationships where we can receive invaluable feedback at critical points of time. When studying for my Master's degree in Human Development Counseling at Vanderbilt University, we learned details about how to best handle a client struggling with suicidal tendencies. We were always told to ask our clients if they had suicidal tendencies and if they had developed a plan to commit suicide. If they answered "yes," they had suicidal tendencies and "yes," they had a plan, we were supposed to ask our client to commit to contacting us prior to following through on their plan to commit suicide. Research on the psychology of suicide has shown that someone is less likely to commit suicide if they are able to open up to someone and share their plan. This is the power of vulnerability and intimate relationships: they can quite literally save our life.

I feel that relationships saved my life during college. I don't know how I could have worked through the panic attacks without having someone to talk to before I went to sleep. Why do we sometimes struggle to open up the most intimate, deep thoughts and emotions we carry with our loved ones? Past experiences, past rejection and experiences of betrayal cause us to hesitate in opening up with people. Sometimes, we struggle with shame about a behavior or thought pattern that we may not want anyone to know about. Shame tries to keep us captive to the behavior, the thought and to our pain, but vulnerability with the right person can free us from this internal battle.

We have all had experiences where we regretted sharing part of our lives with someone. We may have felt in the past that we had "cast our pearls before swine." Sometimes we open up to the wrong person, sometimes we open up at the wrong time and we feel the pain of not only unresolved hurt, but also the pain of feeling misunderstood. Now, we may be left with the regret of sharing our deepest, most hurt self with the wrong person at the wrong time and we feel confused and more hurt.

At the same time that we can fall into the trap of becoming overly introspective, we can also cross a boundary and over share in a desperate attempt to make connection or to ease the pain of a difficult situation.[2] When I was in my 20s, I would waver back and forth between being overly introspective and then crossing boundaries and over sharing in relationships. It can be part of a natural learning curve while we are trying to understand ourselves and connect with others in a deeper way. If this is your first time diving deep into the path of self-awareness and pursuing more intimate relationships, then you may make some mistakes as you learn, but commit to the process and it will be worth it.

In order to be loved, we need people in our lives that know the real us: the us that doesn't always measure up to our own standards, the us that has flaws and weaknesses and the us that fails. Many times, we learn to present a false sense of self to others because of shame and learning to hide out of past experiences of rejection. The reality is that we will never feel loved until we take off the mask and show our true selves to those around us.

Children are beautifully and uniquely themselves. I love watching my son, Cadell Noble play and express himself unhindered. I love seeing my son, Cadell walk up to everyone with utmost confidence that he will be liked saying "hi" with a huge smile on his face. Children, for the most part, don't know how to tune down or play it safe in relationships; they openly share their hearts. Until children experience shame, rejection or emotional pain in relationships, they will continue to be free and unhindered in their expression of love and true identity.

Something happens in childhood that leaves many people marred with the question: "What is wrong with me?" This shame covers the true, unique person and causes the individual to learn to hide their true self out of the fear of rejection. Now, marred by shame, they learn to create a false sense of self, one that is acceptable to the outside world. The more we learn to hide, strive and please others with our false sense of self, the harder it becomes to be known and to experience unconditional love.

Sometimes the hiding is about identity or mistakes and sometimes it is about roles that we play for affirmation and identity. We may judge a role that someone played in our lives which leads to a belief that cripples our identity in the future. In my case, I didn't realize that I had a prejudice against traditional male and female roles in family life until I was married. When I married my husband Eugene, I was thrilled that he enjoyed cooking and that he was actually quite good at it. Also, he didn't mind cleaning and helping with household chores. I found a keeper! However, I was so opposed to traditional female roles that I refused to cook and clean, like ever.

I was dead-set against traditional roles in a marriage that I rebelled against anything that looked somewhat similar to the traditional female/male role. When my husband would come home from work, I would be in my office, deep into my work and most days, I would hardly stop to say, "Hi, welcome home, how was your day?" I would continue to work and make no effort to cook or have a meal with my husband. He would usually figure out what he was going to eat on his own and I would find something to eat on my own or he would cook for us both.

I remember very specifically one time when my husband came home, I was so engrossed in work that I hadn't noticed it was already dark outside. The lights were all off in the house and my husband found me hunched up in front of my computer. Urgently he asked, "Why didn't you turn on any of the lights?" In a daze, I looked up and noticed that the house was dark and foreboding.

A few months later, I was reflecting upon my life one morning when suddenly I saw images flash before my conscious mind: Eugene coming home from work while I continued to work in my office, Eugene cooking and asking for help while I retorted back, "I'm busy working," Eugene getting locked out of the house while I'm having work meetings and he can't get a hold of me because I refused to check my phone during the work day. A dozen or so images flashed before my eyes and I realized something profound in that moment, I had not been prioritizing my marriage at all. Work came first and everything, including my husband, always came last. In an instant, I was back in my childhood watching my mom and dad interact. I see my mom making dinner as she calls us to the door, "Dad's almost home from work, let's go wait for him!" We run outside with our dog, excited to see my dad walking up the stairs of our deck after a long day.

I realized something very deep as I watched the day-to-day images play before my eyes: I made a judgment towards my mom for her choice to be a stay-at-home mom. I concluded, "I don't want to have a traditional marriage with traditional roles, I want to be a career woman." Because of this belief, I was very self-serving in my relationship with my husband. Everything in my marriage revolved around what Eugene could do for me, not what I could do for him. As a child, I didn't realize that there was a genuine interaction of love between my mom and dad, and that my mom made dinner for us every night as an act of love and service. My mom chose to be with us every day as an act of love and prioritizing family over a career. I further realized that I wanted to show love to my spouse, to prioritize our relationship and yes, to even make dinner for him sometimes as an expression of my love.

That day, I wrote my husband a letter and apologized for my selfish ways in our marriage. That fall, we planned a vow renewal in Nashville, Tennessee to recommit to each other. From that point on, we were able to change our relational dynamics to a healthier partnership. However, the change in my behavior did not come until I understood what belief system I developed about marriage in my childhood. How did I discover my belief system about marriage?

First of all, I was a curious observer of my life and I allowed my marriage to be a mirror to reflect back to me things about myself. Secondly, I had a practice of self-reflection where I would journal, meditate and pray. As a result of my self-reflective practices, I began to notice a negative internal monologue about traditional roles in marriage. For example, when my friends who were stay-at-home moms would talk about their struggles, I would judge their lives as boring and monotonous. My thought patterns would be very critical in nature, even deeming their lives not as important as mine.

As a child, we develop our core beliefs through key relationships. When we are relating, interacting and mirroring our caregivers, we naturally make conclusions about the world based upon these interactions. These conclusions can be positive and based upon reality or negative and not based upon reality. If we develop a lot of negative conclusions about the world that are not based upon reality, we will develop a worldview that is skewed. Thus, we begin to experience life differently than other people based upon our unique perception of reality.

In fact, each person on planet earth has developed a unique worldview that will cause him or her to experience life vastly differently than another person. There are clearly some beliefs that are more helpful and more truthful than others. Obviously, making the following conclusion during childhood: "I am rejected and abandoned, and I will always feel alone," will not result in very positive experiences. In fact, this maladaptive core belief will attract more experiences of rejection and abandonment until the belief is challenged. As an adult, we can shift our core beliefs through relationships as we allow our deepest beliefs to surface to our conscious mind to be challenged. Our relationships can be used as a mirror to reflect our inner world in order to help us gain access to limiting belief patterns that we developed throughout childhood.

This is all part of the science of neuroplasticity. Researchers in neuroscience have demonstrated that the brain develops and adjusts throughout a person's lifetime.[3] In fact, cortical remapping is the discovery that the brain continues to create new neural pathways, alters existing ones as it adapts to new experiences, learns new information and creates new memories.[4]

Behavioral researchers identified factors necessary for change.[5] Preparation, planning, action and maintenance are all necessary factors for change to occur and it begins and ends with the neuroplasticity of the brain.[6]

In order to prepare, we need to reflect and grow in self-awareness by adopting journaling and deep-thinking practices. We need to be willing to be brutally honest with others and ourselves in order to examine critical language in our thoughts that are sometimes connected to maladaptive core beliefs. Once you have reflected and discovered critical thought patterns, you are ready for the next step. The next step after reflecting is to confront critical internal monologues that you discover.

I will give you an example from my own life. This is a conversation that would come up sometimes in my marriage, "You expect the house to be clean and food to be on the table when you get home from work. You knew that you were not marrying a stay-at-home wife and mother when we got engaged and nothing has changed! I am not a stay-at-home mom; I am a working mom. It is impossible for me to clean and cook while working on my business during the day!"

I would become very defensive when my husband would have the slightest reaction to the house being a mess or the fact that dinner was not prepared. My reaction would tend to be inappropriate given the context of the relational exchange with my husband. My emotions would become quickly and easily heated as I defended my position as a working mom, not a stay-at-home mom. This is the first clue that you are triggering a maladaptive core belief: inappropriate emotional and verbal responses to family members. Asking questions to reflect and discover the deeper issue can be helpful. For example, reflecting after a fight with your partner: Why did I blow up like that at my spouse? Why am I so emotional right now? What is the deeper issue?

When you reflect on these interactions, you may discover something deeper to a consistent clash in a relationship that is related to a skewed belief system. There are several options about how to move forward with dealing with these patterns. First, find clarity on what the deeper issue is, and try to pinpoint the maladaptive beliefs coming from your critical internal or external monologue. Secondly, you can confront this internal monologue through either journaling or talking out loud to yourself or a trusted friend.

If you choose to write your confrontation, notice your emotions and allow them to be expressed. When I confronted my maladaptive core belief about marriage, I wrote my husband an apology letter, found him that same day and read the letter to him out loud. I was crying as I apologized for how self-serving I had been in our marriage. Everything had been about me up until that point and I was ready to confront my maladaptive belief and change.

My letter to my husband sounded something like this: "Eugene, I am so sorry, I realized something deeply distressing today, I have not been prioritizing our relationship. I have been selfish and self-serving. I think of all the times that you came home from work, excited to see me, but I was too busy working to acknowledge you and the importance of our relationship. You must feel so lonely sometimes in our relationship and it is my fault. I think of all of the times that I didn't acknowledge your needs or the needs of our relationship because of my ambitious pursuits related to my business. Can you forgive me for my selfishness? I want to change and make our relationship a priority."

After I confessed and apologized to my husband, I needed to confront the maladaptive core belief directly. When you confront directly, you can write yourself a letter or you can verbally confront. My verbal confrontation went something like this: "You have not been prioritizing your relationship with your husband. You believe that you cannot be a wife, mother and a businesswoman at the same time. You are stuck in the belief that you have to choose between the three instead of doing all of these roles well. As a child, you watched your mom and dad and you judged their relationship. In fact, you decided that you did not want to be a stay-at-home mother and that you did not want to serve any role similar to that. This judgment that you made is not helping you, as you are not building a strong marriage. In fact, you are sabotaging your marriage right now. It was wrong for you to judge your mom for deciding to be a stay-at-home mom. It was her choice and she did it out of love for you. You are very selfish and critical of others' when their choices do not align with your perspective. You need to release the judgment that you made against your mother and allow yourself to step into your role as a mother and a wife so that your marriage and your relationship with your son can flourish."

After you confront using an emotional tone, you can also confront using a rational tone: "You are wrong about me. There is nothing wrong with me. I am adjusting to being a mom who owns a business and my life is in a good stage. I can be a good wife, mother and business owner. It is possible to fulfill all of my roles and responsibilities without harming one of them. My son needs me to show him love and to be there for him at this stage. I have a unique opportunity to pursue two dreams at the same time and my husband is growing and has a lot of responsibility on his plate. If you make your marriage a priority and learn to value the role of a mother and a wife, you will find more joy in your day to day life."

After you confront critical thought patterns, you disobey the inner voice and don't do what it tells you to do. Be specific in what behavior you are going to stop doing and what behavior you are going to begin doing. I decided to stop working when my husband came home from work and make sure that we had a meal together before I went back to work in my office again. This was a big change and I found that we were both happier when I made this change in behavior.

After you change your behavior, carry out the new behaviors on a daily basis and progressively add in new behaviors as you succeed in the beginning changes. In order to change our behaviors, we need to become aware of maladaptive core beliefs in our subconscious mind and we need to confront, challenge and shift those beliefs. Every action based upon the awareness of the beliefs that we are confronting either strengthens or weakens the connections in the brain. New actions performed over and over again build and strengthen new neural connections in the brain. Emotional connection and awareness in this process is critical as well. Emotions cause neurons to fire and release adrenaline, serotonin and dopamine in the brain, which stimulates change in the brain, helping neurons to become stronger, larger and more complex in their connections.[7] Thus, if we can have emotional awareness and emotional release while we connect with thought patterns and challenge our core beliefs, we will have greater leverage in rewiring our brain.

"Vulnerable love"

Running to my car, I quickly threw my bag in the back, turned the key and stepped on the gas. The sound of metal on metal caused me to cringe and slam on the breaks. What in the world just happened? I looked sharply to my right and I saw that I had just smashed my side mirror into my garage door. Great! Just what I need when I am running late to my internship, I thought to myself. With a sigh of regret and frustration, I pulled forward and continued to back out of my garage, making a mental note to get the side mirror fixed when I head home for Christmas. Oh well, at least my car can still drive, I reflected.

As I began to drive on the highway, the sound of the side mirror flapping against my window caused me to first panic, secondly, to cry and then it prompted me to call my best friend laughing. A ball of emotions began to unravel as I shared the turmoil in my soul from the last few months to my best friend, "This about sums up my life. I try to give my best, show that I care and work hard and it just blows up in my face. I can't believe that I am going to this stupid internship to sit in front of a computer and create teaching materials when I am supposed to be counseling. I can't wait for this to be over."

As I lamented to my best friend, I reflected on the shit-show experience that I had at this internship. A few weeks prior, my mentor and supervising counselor brought me out to lunch in a timid and precarious manner. She had never brought me away from the school to talk; usually we just met in the counseling office. I had been interning at the high school for a few weeks now, learning the ins and outs of being a high school counselor from my supervisor. Up until that point, I had thought that it was going well. Something lingering in the air caused me to sink back into my thoughts and I struggled to catch my breath. I felt my chest tightening and had the same racing thoughts that I had prior to a panic attack. I thought to myself, why is she bringing me to this strange place? All of a sudden, I felt like I was in a horror movie and someone was about to jump out from behind a tree and chop off my head. At least, that would have been less painful than what actually happened.

Awkwardly and suddenly, my supervisor turned her face towards me and half-spoke, half-yelled, "What happened when you were talking with Betsy last week?" Taken aback, I stared back at my supervisor, stunned at the tone of her voice and shaken by the accusatory nature of her tone. I thought back frantically to my interaction with Betsy last week. Betsy shared with me about her friendship woes and how one of her friends talked about her behind her back and the other one deserted her at lunch. I chalked it up to typical 3rd grade drama and insecurities. I listened to her, gave her a treat and walked her back to lunch. Nothing too crazy.

Red flags appeared in my brain when I remembered the short conversation that Betsy and I had as we walked back to the lunchroom. Betsy asked me, "What do I tell my friends when they ask about my conversation with you?" I said the following in a vague sense to not expose the details of our conversation to the world around us, "Just tell them the good things that we talked about and not the bad things." Just as those words escaped my lips, I looked over and saw the librarian peering at me with a strange contemplative look in her eyes. And then I knew. The librarian accused me of something based upon that conversation that I had with Betsy. With a vast array of assumptions that could be pulled from the phrase "just tell them the good things that we talked about and not the bad things," I thought about how insignificant the life of the librarian was and how she probably saw herself as a hero in the plot of a story that simply did not exist.

I sharply breathed as I responded to my supervisor, "Nothing happened in my conversation with Betsy. She was complaining about her friends gossiping behind her back and a few other random 3rd grade issues. She asked me what to tell her friends about our conversation and I told her, "Tell them the good things that we spoke about and not the bad things."

My supervisor peered over at me with the same look of suspicion that I saw on the face of the librarian and I thought to myself, this town is too small, does not have enough going on and they definitely watch too many sci-fi thrillers to do anything good with their brain waves. They wanted drama, so they created drama, and it was going to be about me and the nothingness that happened in my conversation with a 3rd grader complaining about her friends.

The saga that continued from this inconsequential fleeting sentence that was overheard by a desperate, suspicious librarian, would astound most reasonable people. However, here I was, in the midst of the storm of my life, accused of something intangible that I clearly did not do.

No one ever accused me of anything substantial. Rather, the details remained completely elusive and unsubstantial, but you would have thought that I was on trial for murder. First of all, they decided that I couldn't meet with any other students one-on-one for the remainder of my internship as a counselor. What they expected me to do was mind-numbingly confusing. My supervisor at Vanderbilt University came to an immediate meeting with the principal and supervising counselor where they threw around accusatory statements without anything substantial, and I sat there with a deer in headlights look. My supervisor at Vanderbilt was befuddled by my lack of defense, but I really grappled to understand what I was defending myself against. The lofty accusations were so far removed from reality that I struggled to create any substantial defensive posture.

They were so completely wrong about me that I think I was in shock at the absurdity of the whole thing. I also knew I was innocent, and I didn't really have anything to defend. So, I just sat there appalled and shocked by the whole thing.

This easily could have derailed my career as a counselor, made me feel shame and feel like I could not succeed in life. But, I knew that I was a good counselor, and that I did nothing wrong. I would not allow this to leave an impression in my soul about my capabilities as a counselor.

I learned one valuable thing: I sat with my supervisor and teacher from Vanderbilt and she gave me some feedback that was hard to hear, but something that I needed to hear. She said, "You have tremendous presence when you are with people one-on-one. However, you look at people so intensely, so deliberately that it can make some people feel uncomfortable. They may not want to reveal their deepest darkest feelings to you, but the intensity of your gaze makes it feel like you are forcing him or her to open up."

As I sat in the uncomfortable silence and tried to absorb the magnitude of her words, I felt so small and very much misunderstood. I had a lot of compassion for people and I really was motivated out of empathy to try to help, but I was unaware that I had been sabotaging my own best efforts by something like the intensity of my gaze. This was one of those moments. I could run away, far away in my heart from this perspective, deny it and push it away because it hurt like a dagger in the heart; or, I could embrace the pain and allow myself to grow beyond this moment.

Thankfully, I did choose to embrace this painful moment of feedback, and I adjusted my approach. Looking back on my first internship, I realize now that it was one of those defining moments: it was going to make or break me. I believe that it helped to make me who I am today.

There are some things I have learned about myself in the context of relationships that I never could have learned about myself through solitude, journaling, meditation and self-reflection. On the other hand, there are some things that I have learned about myself while journaling, meditating and self-reflecting that I never could have learned about in the context of a relationship. The self-knowledge that I have gained in the context of relationships tends to be more humbling and painful than what I discover about myself in the context of solitude.

I have a tendency towards perfectionism and using perfectionism to cover up shame. In the situation of the internship, it was so emotionally painful that I had to open up to people around me to find emotional relief. The love and acceptance of my friends in the moment of my deepest shame allowed me to love myself through the betrayal of false accusation. In fact, I learned that flaws and weaknesses are the way in which we receive grace and learn to love us despite our shortcomings and failings (even though, ironically, I had done nothing wrong at my internship).

However, I had the opportunity to integrate myself more fully and to have my internal and external personas become more unified. Integrity is met when a soul is fully integrated and has no differences between the external and internal self. In a state of integrity, the person we are inside is perfectly reflected externally to those around us. Prior to the false accusations at the high school, I didn't realize that I had intensity in my gaze that was freaking people out. I thought that I was exhibiting a great sense of compassion for humanity, not prying into people's souls against their will. If the false accusations never came up at that internship, there would have been no reason for my supervising counselor to give me the feedback that I needed to change in order to become a better version of myself.

Vulnerability can bring fear because we may engage in a behavior that pushes love away. Further, we may receive feedback that hurts in the moment when we have close relationships, but we will have an opportunity to change in order to become more fully integrated.

The questions are: 1. Do you allow people close enough? 2. Are you humble enough to receive the feedback you need from that relationship? 3. Are you vulnerable enough to allow the feedback to change you? Most of us stand at a distance, close enough to not feel completely alone, yet far enough away to not get pricked by feedback that we don't want to hear. As Theodore Roethke stated, "Love is not love until love is vulnerable." Most people just play the part of love, but don't let people in close enough to be vulnerable to them and to be in a position of being hurt, betrayed or rejected. Can you let love into your failings, shortcomings and unlovable parts? Can you let love be vulnerable?

Section 2: Relationships Reflect Me: What Do You See?

Chapter 5: The Art of Developing True Intimacy

Middle school invited a special type of torture to my life that made me sensitive to rejection years after the fact. I remember the battleground of middle school being the lunchroom. The queasy, insecure fear of, "Who am I going to sit with today?" always appeared as I entered the lunchroom. I knew the tables that were off-limits to me and pretty much everyone else; the cool table welcomed the popular and the beautiful. And then there was the athletic, funny and smart table that I had an unofficial "alternate" seat to. There were 3 of us who would rotate the last seat of the athletic, funny and smart table, and I never knew which day the seat would be open to me and which day the seat would be closed to me. It brought much anxiety and a desire to perform and fit their "community standards." Some days, I didn't even feel like trying, and I would find myself in the bathroom stall with my lunch, crying silently.

It all sounds very dramatic and I'm sure that most of my lunchroom woes are true; however, middle school with all of the awkwardness of glasses or not, braces or not, the right clothes, the right personality and the right look all brought shame and rejection that some would struggle to recover from. On the other hand, it was also the beginning stages of budding friendships in which some have lasted until today.

During middle school, amidst all of the rejection and fear of rejection, I remember developing a really large and grotesque wart. I had it treated at the dermatologist and went with my friends to the lake on the weekend. After the treatment, the wart grew to the size of a small egg on my big toe. My friends thought that the wart was gross and yet really funny at the same time and in a mocking and slightly endearing manner, my nickname became "Egg." My friends still sometimes call me Egg, and it actually brings back fond memories now even though it was horrifying at the time.

These awkward and weird moments are sometimes how people feel every time they try to share themselves in a real way to their friends and family. At some point, some people learn to not share or reveal too much out of a fear of rejection. However, alone and isolated, we have an ability to deceive ourselves and create false images of ourselves. Intimacy rescues us from our fantasy world and introduces us to ourselves: the good, the bad and the ugly. The relationships closest to us can help us to grow and become better people if we are willing to see our warts and treat them to the best of our ability. If we continue to hide in shame and keep ourselves from the people closest to us, we will evade the depth of intimacy needed to bring transformation to our souls.

Imagine what it would be like to live your whole life and never be known by anyone? How would you feel? And how can someone know you when you don't know yourself? Independence is an illusion that prevents us from entering deeply into relationships. We have a deep-seated fear that if people knew the real us, they wouldn't love us. And yet, I always remember being at the lake with my friends when the wart had grown to the size of an egg. Yes, it was gross and yes it was an awkward social moment when they started to call me "Egg." However, I actually started to feel more accepted and part of the group after having the nickname, "Egg" thrust upon me. And I think that my friends started to like me more after they saw my wart. They could relax at the reality that I was imperfect and flawed too, just like them.

We want to be loved, but we hold back, thinking that we will be judged and rejected by the people closest to us. In most cases, the things that you thought would cause people to stop loving you actually lead them to love you more. I would rather experience rejection when trying to establish intimacy than to feel completely alone in the world. When we feel alone, we struggle with the belief that life is hard for me, but why does everyone else seem to have it all together? We can fall into traps of addiction that disconnect us from reality and attempt to affirm that we are the center of our own universe.

If you want to experience true intimacy and oneness in a relationship physically, emotionally, intellectually and spiritually, you need to learn to get comfortable with your quirks and warts. Most people have not fully accepted themselves; thus, they are limited in what they are comfortable sharing with loved ones. When we relegate certain topics as private and controversial, we can slowly become a closed tomb of boring factual information.

Relationships can either be consuming too much of our identity or not enough of our identity. When we have misplaced priorities, relationships either become the most important aspect of our lives or the least important aspect of our lives. In the past, I have fallen into the trap of trying to use relationships to fix me and to fill an endless void in my soul. I still remember the day that I was journaling and meditating in my townhouse when I heard the phrase, "Joe is an idol." I was quite shocked and stood straight up in my chair. Joe was my best friend, I shared everything with him and I believed that we would be together for the rest of our lives. What could this possibly mean?

All of a sudden, Joe was at the door, asking to take me to Starbucks that night to "talk." The words that I heard during my meditation time began to haunt me. At Starbucks, my worst fears were confirmed when Joe broke up with me even though we weren't dating. He wanted to "lay the relationship down." It was one of the most excruciating things that I had experienced emotionally up until that point because we had become so close. All of a sudden, we were not communicating, and I felt like all of my emotional stability left with Joe. I became a rollercoaster of emotions and felt like I was drowning in a quicksand of despair, depression and loneliness. It was clear at that point that Joe had become everything to me: my main and only priority in life in which everything and everyone else revolved.

I needed to get it together, seriously. I had to rebuild and refocus my time and energy on other relationships. Over time, the experience was balancing and helpful to my overall maturity and growth. Using a relationship as a bandage over past wounds and pain is not very effective. Nor is allowing one person to be THE stabilizing force in your life.

To have a deep oneness in our relationships, we need to work on the depth of 4 different types of intimacy: intellectual intimacy, spiritual intimacy, emotional intimacy and physical intimacy. Intellectual intimacy is more than simply knowing what a person thinks about a given topic. Intellectual intimacy is knowing how a person thinks, why they have come to certain conclusions, what drives them as an individual, what inspires and motivates their ideas. It becomes helpful to view your role as a curious observer in your main relationship to look beyond the opinion itself in order to understand what caused your partner to believe that an idea is good, true, noble and just.[1] Intellectual intimacy blossoms in a non-judgmental environment.

The second type of intimacy that we can develop is spiritual intimacy. The beginning stage of spiritual intimacy is deciding on the essential purpose of our relationship: Why are we together? To live a life full of purpose and passion, you need to explore how your main relationship can help you to become the best version of yourself. Our relationship will have room to breathe and develop if we give space for us to be wrong, to not get what we want all of the time and to seek understanding instead of placing blame onto the other person. Spiritual intimacy can grow when we have established the purpose and mission of our relationship that goes beyond raising children. Spiritual intimacy can flourish if we can talk about spiritual concerns, ask each other spiritual questions to understand our differing perspectives, pray together and develop habits of gratitude and forgiveness together.

The third type of intimacy that we can develop in our relationship is emotional intimacy. Developing emotional intimacy takes humility, vulnerability and a level of emotional intelligence. Emotional intelligence can be developed through self-reflection, journaling and meditation. In a relationship that has deep emotional intimacy, we value revealing ourselves in a healthy way and sharing our emotions in a way that allows us to deepen our connection.

The fourth type of intimacy in the relationship with a spouse or partner is physical intimacy. Physical intimacy is easy and can be manipulated. It can also be used to fill the void of intimacy in the other 3 types of intimacy. Physical intimacy brings oneness in the relationship, but it can be a detriment to our ability to develop intimacy in the future if we have multiple sexual partners. Each time we have a sexual relationship, we become one. But when oneness is established multiple times, our souls become fragmented and oneness in other forms of intimacy becomes more challenging as a result. We can be disorientated after a sexual relationship with another person has ended. Each sexual relationship claims a piece of our soul and causes us to become more fragmented in our soul realm.

Matthew Kelly, in his book, *The Seven Levels of Intimacy,* writes about the different levels of intimacy and how to deepen intimacy in relationships. If you want to fully understand the seven levels, I suggest that you read his book in its entirety. I will briefly review the seven levels that he describes so that you can apply them to your closest relationships.[2]

The first level of relationships is the cliché. This is a casual interaction with only superficial exchanges and is commonly used in daily interactions with strangers. However, sometimes our main relationships can be diminished to superficial, one or two words answers. For example, if you ask your partner, "What did you do today?" And they respond by saying: "The same old stuff." This is a cliché response that blocks further questions and a deeper interaction.

How do you move beyond the 1st level of intimacy? By spending quality time together with no agenda, you can move beyond the level of a cliché relationship. Start with 2 hours, 1 time per week spending concentrated quality time together where there is no time pressure or agenda. After you have a regular time once a week where you connect in this manner, you can add one whole day together once a month and a weekend getaway once a quarter.

The 2nd level of intimacy is factual. This is communication that focuses solely on the facts: daily events, weather, what you did, sports and what's happening in the world. This also keeps the interaction from being too intimate and avoids any potential conflict. Facts are useful when you are getting to know someone, but it is not the main way to relate with those closest to us if we want any depth of relationship. Our core relationships need to move past the events of the day or the facts that are black and white.

The path that leads to intimacy is blocked to those who are unwilling to practice non-judgment. When we judge a person for their past, appearance and how they live their life, there is no openness to get to know them past the stereotypes that we have created in our mind. Try this simple exercise: for the next 24-hours try not to judge a single person or situation. Instead, give people the benefit of the doubt and seek understanding in why people say or do things. This type of non-judgment fosters open and honest communication. Judgment kills relationships.

Just as judgment kills relationships, gossip kills relationships. When we talk idly about people in a way that destroys their character or that sheds negative light on them, we sabotage any opportunity to have a good relationship with the person we are talking about. Further, the person hearing the gossip will develop a false understanding of the person being gossiped about which will end up marring their relationship with the person as well. Gossip quite literally separates friendships and relationships and is like poison to a relationship.

I had a close relationship with a friend who had a habit of gossiping often to me about other people. It caused a wedge in our relationship because I had a hard time trusting this friend to not also talk about me to other people. Further, the people she talked about with me were people that I did not know very well. I found it impossible to get to know them after I heard so many intimate details about their past from my friend. It was quite disheartening because I did not want to engage in gossip. At a certain point in my friendship, I had to write a letter to my friend to express my hurt and frustrations surrounding her manner of speech towards other people. Over time, my friend realized that she did struggle with gossip and that she wanted to end her habit of gossiping. We have a much better relationship now and I don't feel uncomfortable in interactions with her because she doesn't gossip anymore.

To diffuse gossip, you can learn to say the following phrases after someone shares intimate details about another person:

- "Perhaps we don't have all of the facts."

- "Perhaps we should discuss this next time when we are with Becky so that she can tell us what happened."
- "I think that we should give Becky the benefit of the doubt."
- "I have also done things in my life that I wish I had not"
- "I will never forget how Becky made a meal train for me after my son died, it was so generous and kind of her."

If you have a friend that has a habit of gossiping often, you may have to confront them more directly like I did with my friend. This can be done in a loving and gentle way. I find that writing letters to confront loved ones helps me to express my deeper thoughts and emotions without feeling so vulnerable and intimidated by the possibility of conflict.

In the 3rd level of intimacy, we share our opinions. This is the first place in intimacy where conflict and disagreement can occur when people don't agree on a given topic. In fact, some people learn to stop sharing their opinions in an attempt to avoid conflict. However, this diminishes an intimate connection. To know someone fully, it's important to be free to share your opinions with one another. Over time, some people develop conversational strategies to avoid certain topics because of the sensitive nature of the topic. For example, when someone brings up a controversial opinion, someone can tell a joke, use sarcasm, change the subject and force the conversation back to a comfortable place with less vulnerability. We can quite literally train people to not bring up certain topics in conversation.

Part of maturation of self and maturation of relationships is the ability to be at peace in the company of people who hold different opinions. To be able to hold a lively debate or a healthy discussion with someone you don't agree with takes wisdom, self-awareness and emotional intelligence. Most people are not able to participate in a lively debate without feeling the pressure to convert the other person to hold their personal beliefs on a given topic. Are we so unsure of our own opinions that we feel threatened by people who have opposing views?

If we have a common goal and purpose in our relationship, many arguments can be avoided. Most people spend the majority of their time trying to convince the other person of their point of view. To move to a place of maturity in relationships, we need to accept that we will not agree on every topic. In a mature relationship, both parties choose to not judge the other's opinion, and act as curious observers to understand how and why each person has come to a different conclusion than the other on the same topic. Many times, the conflict can be a clash of personal goals and worldviews. In a primary relationship with a partner or a spouse, it can be helpful to agree on the purpose of the relationship. One purpose that can be helpful is to help each other become the best versions of us. If we start with this common purpose in mind, it brings everything else into proper perspective and allows our partner freedom to be their self while giving the relationship room to breathe.

The art of genuine agreement is to start by seeking to establish common ground in a conversation. A person who knows how to develop mature relationships will seek to find agreement in the midst of a topic where there may be conflicting views. Many people start a conversation where the disagreement lies. The goal of authentic discussion is to explore a certain subject, not necessarily to be right or to win a debate. Simply work on exploring the path that brought the other person to his or her opinion and try to understand their vantage point. Are there any circumstances where the other person may be right? Try to be open to new ideas, and never shut yourself off from the possibility that you are wrong on a given topic.

We need to learn to disagree in a graceful manner in order to maintain the dignity and respect of a relationship. Every opinion says something about who we are. Our opinions reveal our core values, expectations and beliefs. If we can respect differing opinions and remain dedicated to a common search for truth, we can avoid unnecessary arguments. Keep the following in mind: it isn't your job to fix the relationship; however, it is the job of the relationship to fix you. To show respect, we can accept that, quite simply, people have developed their own opinions based upon their unique experiences. Opinions are constantly evolving. The core of a person is not the sum of their beliefs and opinions. Rather, a person is much more than this. To understand someone, we need to start with respect and acceptance. To accept someone fully, we have to allow him or her to be themselves rather than trying to make them who we want them to be. Surrender control and the rights to fix or change the other person. Allow your relationship to be a mirror in which you make changes to your own view, beliefs and character. This way, both people in the relationship begin to become the best versions of themselves in full autonomy, and yet in a quest for oneness.

In the fourth level of intimacy, according to Matthew Kelly, we share our hopes and dreams with our significant other. This level says something about how we want to live our lives and the person we want to become in the future. Our hidden self emerges in our dreams for the future.

The first step in this level of intimacy is to develop your personal sense of identity, which we explored in **Chapter 4: Embracing Your Eccentricity**. We need to explore our identity and discover what makes us come alive, as this will define our hopes for the future. The next step is revealing your future desires and dreams to your partner. We tend to reveal our dreams to people who accept us without judgment.

If this level of intimacy proves to be challenging, it may be that you need to define your identity further, and discover what makes you unique. I remember vividly when my husband Eugene and I first started to date, we would talk for hours about our hopes and dreams for the future. After being married and having children, day-to-day stressors of life can sometimes suffocate dreams. My husband and I continually re-center our lives towards the achievement of long-term dreams. We make small steps towards the life that we want to live long-term as the process of achieving dreams takes time and patience.

We recently launched Noble International, a non-profit, that will fund restoration homes in Cape Town for at-risk youth. As of 2021, our non-profit is funding a feeding program in an impoverished area that we want to impact in a deeper way long-term. We have also made steps towards caring for 24 orphans in Uganda. We are making small steps towards our global vision and the project will eventually unfold to its full potential.

In order to build an intimate relationship with our significant other, our relationship needs space to breathe so that hopes and dreams can manifest. Being aware of the dreams the people you love carry is just as important as being aware of the dreams that you have for your life. Are we going to help each other fulfill our long-term dreams? The dreams that we hold are part of the vision that molds our lives as well as our relationship with one another.

The big difference between my relationship with Joe and my relationship with my now husband, Eugene, is the commonality of our dreams. Joe and I had a deep emotional and intellectual connection and we understood each other. However, we did not share the same long-term vision for our lives, and this is where our relationship ultimately broke down. For a relationship to last long-term, our dreams for our future need to align and act as a rudder to keep our relationship on track to where we want to land in the future. Many relationships lack the long-term vision that helps a relationship go through the struggles that all relationships have. I can endure a lot when I see the end picture of where we are heading. I can't endure much when I don't envision a hope for my future with someone.

When Eugene and I started dating, he told me that his visa was going to expire and that we should not date seriously. I, however, told him straightforward, "I can travel." Our relationship energized dreams in my heart to travel and work with non-profit mission projects, which helped me to find the next piece of my identity puzzle. Dreams bring passion and life to a relationship that not much else can emulate.

I love the movie, *The Pursuit of Happiness*, except for one part. One part of the movie bothers me because it is an accurate depiction of most relationships at a certain point. Will Smith's character was struggling to sell devices that would act like an MRI for doctors. He decided instead to start pursuing an internship on Wall Street to learn how to become a stockbroker. His partner scoffed at him and mocked him, as she did not believe in him anymore. She was tired of the financial pressure and struggle to make it as a couple and she simply wanted to quit. At one point, Will Smith's character said in frustration, "Do you want to leave? You're weak, you're weak." And they break up right before Will Smith's character finds the big breakthrough that changes his life. If she just would have stuck it out 1 more year, she would have reaped the reward of the struggle, but she couldn't endure the process of delayed gratification. She had become resentful and no longer believed in the vision of her husband. So many relationships end in the mundane frustrations of life. If, however, the relationship had an overarching purpose that it was pursuing, many would find a way through the day-to-day struggles.

The path to realize the dream is not glamorous, it is not for the weak; rather, it is for the couple who have a vision that they will not surrender, even when it seems impossible. Our success in any area of our life depends upon our character and our ability to delay gratification, apply discipline and patiently wait for the manifestation for which we hope.

My husband and I have been on a journey of many years to establish our non-profit, Noble International. We have been through many intense battles along the way. Our son, Noble Thomas died during labor and delivery in 2016 and the trauma was tremendous and beyond anything I had ever endured. We desire to see good come out of our tragic loss and have started to build Noble's legacy through Noble International.

Do you have a dream that is worth the sacrifice and delayed gratification that it will take to accomplish it? If we are only interested in fulfilling personal desires for pleasure and instant gratification, we may abort the dreams and passions that first ignited our lives as a couple. Dreams bring clarity and focus to a relationship.

In the fifth level of intimacy, we learn to share our true feelings with our significant other. There are several dimensions to growing in emotional intimacy with our significant other. First of all, emotional intimacy depends upon our ability to identify and express our emotions to another person. How can we share our emotions when we are unaware of their existence? This is something that many people struggle to express within a relationship and need to develop emotional intelligence. The ability to emotionally connect in relationships hinges upon our individual process of emotional awareness.

The next step is equally challenging. We need to learn how, when and where to reveal our feelings with our spouse. Sometimes we know how we feel and we attempt to share our feelings, but we are shot down because we share at a time that is stressful and there is no space for our significant other to connect with our emotions.

Our emotions reveal our brokenness, our humanity and our vulnerability. If we all had 1 or more genuinely intimate relationships where we could reveal our true feelings, we may not need therapists. Revealing our emotions can feel like a risk when we are unsure how our loved one will receive us. Timing is everything in revealing emotions. If my husband is hungry, stressed or working, it is the wrong time to reveal my deepest feelings. I will end up feeling emotionally abandoned and say something like, "This made it worse. I should not have told you how I feel." When we need to have intimate conversations with our significant other, we can learn to create space and the right timing by saying something like, "I really need to have a few minutes to talk and share with you today." This allows the other person to pick the right time.

In an accepting relationship, we feel free to share our emotions without the fear of being judged harshly. If we are afraid of being criticized, we may not share how we truly feel. If you can accept your loved one for who they are, try not to change them, they can respond by opening up how they feel. Feelings change and are momentary, but having a safe space to share our feelings within the context of a relationship will make a difference over time.

There are several reasons why your relationship may lack emotional intimacy. First of all, if we do not listen to our significant other in a way that allows them to open up, then they may not feel safe to share their feelings. Many times, when two people are engaged in a discussion, the other person focuses on formulating the next thing that they want to say instead of truly listening and connecting with the other person's experience and emotions. Ask questions, repeat back what you think you heard and ask for clarity in case you missed their perspective. There is value in learning to listen in a way that allows someone to describe his or her inner world. I still remember a note someone wrote to me that said the following, "After talking to you, I feel like I know and understand myself better. Thank you for listening to me." It is still one of the best compliments that I have ever received.

When was the last time that you made your loved one feel like nothing else matters in the world but him or her? As you tune into your own inner world and draw out the inner world of your partner, you will find an emotional connection that deeply anchors your relationship through stormy times.

In the sixth level of intimacy, we share our faults, fears and failures with our significant other. This is when we examine the wounds of our past in the context of an intimate relationship. We expose ourselves until we are emotionally naked in front of our loved one. Some believe this level of intimacy is only appropriate for a primary relationship. However, some have friends with whom they are comfortable bearing their soul to as well.

After the tragic loss of our son, Noble Thomas, my husband and I shared the deepest level of emotional intimacy we have ever experienced in our relationship. We shared a deeply traumatic experience together and it defined our relationship in a positive way. After Noble died, we were able to open up deeper fears, wounds and pain to each other in a way that we had not been able to previously. I remember months after Noble died being terrified every time my phone rang because I thought that it was news of the death of another loved one. I was terrified because I knew that in my fragile emotional state, I could not handle more grief. I was able to share these fears with my husband, Eugene, and we became closer while we learned to rely upon each other emotionally.

Further, I remember making travel plans to South Africa to share about the life of Noble with Eugene's family. Eugene shared with me a strange sensation he felt while we made travel plans. He felt that I was going to be abducted on our trip. We both had many irrational fears while we grieved the loss of our son, but these moments bonded us together.

Fear is more than an emotion because when we are operating in fear, we can be driven to make decisions that are irrational. Processing our fears with our significant other can diminish the impact of fear and its innate ability to steer our decisions towards impulsivity and irrationality. When we operate in a state of fear, we bulldoze over our intuition and stop listening to ourselves. We also lack the mental capacity to logically think through a decision.

In this level of intimacy, we own up to our past mistakes, faults and habits that have diminished our true sense of self and we invite our partner into helping us change for the better. If I am unable to say, I made these mistakes in the past, then it may also be hard for me to admit when I am wrong in the present. Instead of being a victim, we can take ownership of our past and make decisions towards a better future. Are we going to continue to let our past determine our future or are we going to make choices that will allow our future to be different than our past?

In one moment, we express the best version of ourselves and in the next moment, we can abandon our ideals. Intimacy is meant to help bring freedom from the ways that we distort reality and deceive ourselves.

Relationships expose the maladaptive beliefs that govern our subconscious mind if we allow our partner close enough for our maladaptive beliefs to become apparent.

Most alcoholics try to hide that they have a problem and in hiding, the addiction dominates their mind and soul. When an alcoholic admits he or she has a problem, this is the beginning of freedom from shame and an opportunity to walk into a new path. When we bring our issues into a loving relationship, they begin to work themselves out.

Because of what Eugene and I endured together, our relationship became deeper and we were able to move from level five intimacy to level six one year after Noble died. When we share our faults with our significant other, the intimate relationship can be a catalyst to challenge our belief system, which can lead to a change in our behaviors. As I shared in the previous chapter, I opened up to Eugene about the fact that I failed to prioritize my marriage over my career. Because I understood why I prioritized my career over my family, I was able to deal with the root cause: my faulty belief system. Undoing the judgment that I made towards my mom's choice to be a stay-at-home mom, I was free to develop a new belief system regarding marriage and family life. I could then make new decisions of how to engage with my husband and my son.

In the seventh level of intimacy, we learn to help each other fulfill our legitimate needs in a dynamic collaboration. At this moment, our quest to know and be known turns into a real partnership. We all have legitimate needs in the physical, emotional, intellectual and spiritual realm. When we have what we need in each area, we will start to thrive.

When legitimate needs are chronically unmet, we become irritable, restless, discontented and frustrated. Collaborating in the most dynamic way is when we learn to create a lifestyle with the person we love that is focused on both of our legitimate needs being fulfilled. This will cause our partner and our relationship to thrive.

In the seventh level of intimacy, we are at the pinnacle of our quest for intimacy. We can be vulnerable and show our needs to one another. In an authentic relationship, you would never take pleasure in selfish fulfillment at the expense of the other person. In a mature relationship, where both people are in a purposeful partnership and want the best for each other, the seventh level of intimacy can be accomplished.

After I graduated from college, my mom, dad and I traveled to Italy to watch the winter Olympics. It was a tradition growing up for my mom and I to be glued to the Olympic figure skating competitions. I grew up figure skating and we loved the sport. We had a great trip with so many wonderful memories and experiences. At one point, we were traveling between five small cities in Italy and we were running late to board a train to the next city. If we missed the train, we would be stuck for a minimum of 3 hours waiting for the next train. The city was so small that we had already seen all of it. We needed to make our train.

Finishing lunch, we headed to the train station that was several yards away. We thought that it would be a simple transaction. Much to our surprise, we arrived to where the train station was supposed to be and there was a spiral staircase that winded down for several flights before reaching the main platform. Further, once you reached the platform, the booth to purchase your tickets was another 800 meters away with a tunnel that led to where we needed to be to board the train. In a split second, we realized that we were in trouble and about to miss our train. We took off running as fast as we could down the stairs. As soon as we hit the platform, we started sprinting towards the booth to purchase our tickets. My dad took the lead, I was a close second and my mom started trailing behind. We realized that we were really in trouble as we heard the train whistle blow, signaling that it was almost to the station.

As we started sprinting even faster, my dad shouted while laughing, "Every man for himself!" We all started laughing as we were running. My dad and I made it to the booth, purchased our tickets and ran down the tunnel to get to the other side where we could board the train. At that point, we visibly saw the train only 800 yards away. My mom was still on the other side of the tunnel as my dad and I arrived to where we could board the train. We looked over the train tracks to my mom and saw her wide-eyed, in a panic, looking wildly from the train, the tunnel and finally to where we were standing. She would not have sufficient time to run down the tunnel to get to the other side where we were and still make the train. In a split second, my mom jumped into the train tracks and ran across the tracks in front of the train. My dad pulled her up safely to the platform just in time. Seconds later, the train pulled up next to us and we jumped into the train. We were laughing so hard that we started to cry, not noticing all of the people on the train glaring at us in distaste and shame. You could almost read their thoughts, "Stupid Americans, you could have died running in front of that train...this is not funny, shame on you."

That moment ended up being the best memory of our trip, one that we still bring up and laugh about. My mom still scoffs at the fact that my dad shouted out the phrase, "every man for himself" as she trailed behind us. On a serious note, "every man for himself," seems to be almost an American mantra. The average American household seems to be a chaotic stream of individual pursuits with no common, collective agenda guiding the family unit. If we stay in the mentality of "every man for himself," setting ourselves against one another in a competition where there is only one winner, we will continually engage in battles between conflicting agendas wielding manipulation and control as a weapon against those we love.

Relationships are not about getting what you want; relationships are about helping each other become the best versions of us. Can you set aside your individual desires and come together with your partner to focus on everyone's legitimate needs getting met in the family? Love is choosing, desiring and pursuing to see everyone fulfilled in the pursuit of becoming the best version of himself or herself. Love is willing to lay down our personal agenda for the good of the relationship. Are you willing to suffer for love? If you are not willing to pay the price, you will not develop the dynamic collaboration and deepest place of intimacy. We need to hone our ability to recognize the needs of those we love.

The seventh level of intimacy requires sacrifice to become one cohesive unit. It is a culmination of all that we have discovered about each other through the other levels of intimacy. We can form a collective ego and now the real journey begins. If we as two individuals can create a lifestyle based upon mutual fulfillment of legitimate needs, our deepest level of intimacy bonds our fates as one.

Now, take some time to explore the questions and exercises in the companion workbook. Some of these exercises will include your significant other. If you do not have a spouse or significant other, you can do some of the exercises with a best friend or family member, where appropriate.

Section 3: Unraveling the Imprint of Trauma

Chapter 1: The Dream-Like State of Surviving Trauma & How to Move Past Surviving into Thriving

Startled, I hear my phone ring loudly next to me in the car. As I look at the caller-ID, I feel my heart sink and my chest tighten. A battle ensues in my head of whether or not I should answer the call. I have a sinking feeling that the call will surface another tragedy that I simply cannot emotionally handle. I decide to answer the call after wrestling with the decision internally for several seconds. "Hello…is everything okay?" I quickly ask for the bad news to get it over with as fast as possible.

My pulse jumps through the roof and I can't catch a breath as I wait for the answer. "Everything is fine, just calling to check on you." My mom answers calmly. The feelings of impending doom escape from my lips as I take a sharp breath out and try to relax my body.

Later that evening, my husband comes home from work and I ask him sharply, "Hey, do you feel anxious every time someone calls you, like there might be another tragedy?" I'm curious to know if I am the only one dangling on the edge of insanity. My husband looks at me thoughtfully and then nods his head in agreement; "You know what, now that you say that, I do feel nervous when people call. I just didn't pinpoint it to what happened with Noble. It must be connected."

As long as someone else feels as crazy as I do, I feel slight relief in my chest, affirmed in my daily emotional struggle to simply answer my phone. Memories of the previous months flood my mind as I think back to what brought me to the edge of sanity. I watch as if seeing someone else's life flash before my mind's eye, the events that proceeded and followed the death of my first child, Noble Thomas.

Everyone responds differently to trauma depending upon their life experiences, their current worldview and their personal perception of the trauma. Trauma imprints real changes in the wiring of the brain, the stress response system and the overall biochemistry of the body. Trauma that is unresolved alters the threat perception system in the brain.[1] Thus, my "irrational" fears of another tragic event occurring was completely normal; my threat perception system was amped up because the trauma of losing Noble was yet to be fully resolved in my mind, heart and body.

My grandma had died just 2 weeks prior to Noble Thomas Van Zyl coming and going so quickly. At the end of my pregnancy, my grandma's death and funeral hardly registered, as I was so overwhelmed. Then, my son died during labor and delivery. I remember feeling completely numb about my grandmother's death after Noble died. I still don't think I grieved the loss of my grandma because of how overwhelmed with grief I was after Noble died. After trauma, it is common to experience irrational reactions, intense emotions and numbness. These reactions occur when the trauma remains in the unresolved stage. Each step forward into the grieving process, I focused on sensing, identifying and releasing my intense emotions so that I could resolve the trauma of losing a child.

My days seemed to come and go in a dream-like state. Many times after trauma, the dorsolateral prefrontal cortex (DLPFC) becomes deactivated. This part of the brain helps us to feel centered in time. With the deactivation of the DLPFC, trauma victims lose their sense of past, present and future.[2] I definitely felt like I was floating through time, and my daily experiences seemed unconnected, meaningless and vague.

After trauma, some victims experience something called Post-traumatic Stress Disorder or PTSD. Flashbacks or memories of the trauma can occur at any moment, day or night, and propels the trauma victim into deep, intense feelings of grief. While the trauma is replayed over and over again, stress hormones engrave memories more deeply into the mind. During this process, day-to-day events are monotonous, tedious and aggravating as it becomes impossible for someone in a state of trauma to feel fully alive with joy and purpose.

Flashes of memories appeared at unforeseen moments in my day-to-day life. Over time, the story line became more and more defined and I could piece together a beginning, middle and end to the story of Noble dying during labor and delivery. The story goes something like this:

I am drawing a bath, waiting for labor pains to ramp up again after having some reprieve from the labor pains that ebbed and flowed throughout the night. Next, I call my husband to tell him to come home from work so that we can leave for the birthing center. We arrive at the birthing center and the nurse checks my pulse and blood pressure before examining me to decide if I am dilated enough to stay. It was my first baby and everyone seems slightly hesitant about my ability to stay and have a baby that day. The expectation is that I am still in pre-labor and that I may need to go home and wait it out some more.

A sigh of relief escapes my lips when the nurse says to me, "You can stay! You are dilated at a 5.0." I feel relief run through my entire body. Something is finally happening after waiting for weeks for labor to start. I thought to myself many times that the due date was wrong and that this baby should be here by now. Impatience in the process made my last 3 weeks of pregnancy almost unbearable besides that fact that I gained 3 times the weight that most people gain during pregnancy.

I desired to birth in the birthing pool, so I eagerly wait, as they draw the water for me to enter and start the next phase of labor. I am completely caught off guard by the unavoidable labor pains that seem to possess my entire body, making it impossible to do anything but try to take deep breaths in between. There is not a thought towards the entire cooler full of food that we packed. Except for the time that my husband tries to grab a snack quickly while I yell at him, "What are you doing? I need you!" We clearly did not know what we were getting into prior to arriving at the birthing center. At another point during labor and delivery, my husband tries to coordinate his breath with mine and I hear his voice singing along with my deep moans, irritated, I yell at him, "Stop it! You sound too happy!" The nurses, doula and midwife try to hide their looks of glee and laughter at the common scene playing before them of a husband and wife missing each other during labor and delivery.

It feels like time stands still and then all of a sudden, one of the nurses proclaims in triumph, "I see some hair! You are starting to crown! It will be any moment now!" I again feel relief, but troubled that I am getting tired. I cannot imagine how this baby is going to come out of my body. The expectation of a swift delivery after crowning is dashed as the labor pains continue in intensity and never seem to let up. The baby's head shows no signs of movement.

Two hours later, I am desperate for relief; I feel an odd sense of panic, confusion and doom. Something is wrong. I attempt to utter phrases of "something is wrong, he won't come out" in-between pushing and breathing, but I struggle to communicate fully the depths of my despair and fear. I intuitively know that something is terribly wrong. The nurses ask if I would try to stand outside of the tub to push and see if gravity helps. As soon as I stand outside of the tub, I am in shock and horrific pain. I want to immediately go back into the water. It feels wrong to be outside of the tub. After pushing outside of the tub a few times, I convince them to let me back into the tub. I gave up trying to tell them something was wrong. It was my first baby, what do I know?

As soon as I enter the tub, they check for baby's heartbeat again as they had been doing in between each time I had pushed. Suddenly, the nurse cannot find the heartbeat. The atmosphere in the room shifts in an instant. I hear the midwife say urgently, "Get on the bed; we need to do an episiotomy." I quickly move out of the tub and onto the bed and everything picks up to warp speed as the energy completely shifts towards a medical intervention. The midwife cuts me and the baby is easily pushed out. Immediately, the nurses start CPR on my baby, as he is visibly blue. In a panic, we start to call for our baby to come back to us and pray for God to intervene.

Initially, we thought that our baby was a girl. We had decided to wait and find out the gender at the time of birth. As we call to our baby with a girl name, the nurses quickly tell us, "It's a baby boy." In shock, I switch the name to our boy name, saying, "Noble Thomas come back to us now, we love you." Time seems to speed up and slow down all at the same time as the ambulance arrives with the paramedics, whisking my baby away. I tell my husband to leave and go with our baby as I am getting stitched up and need to be stable before leaving the birthing center.

In my mind, I feel calm and relieved. I feel a strong sense that everything will be okay. They will revive my son and we will go home together soon. I call my mom and dad and tell them what happened, my mom moans, "No, no, no…" as I tell her that they rushed my baby to the NICU. I call my pastor and tell him the same thing, "Please meet Eugene and my parents at the hospital."

A half an hour or so passes and the nurses ask me if I want to take a shower prior to leaving. "No," I decline, "I don't have time to take a shower, I have to go and find my baby." My dad picks me up at the birthing center in order to bring me to the hospital. He cries in the car as I get in saying, "I don't know how to tell you this, but your baby is dead." The words float away in the distance and simply do not register in my brain. "Take me to him. I need to see him," I say in a monotone voice. In my mind, it wasn't true. He was alive. I am going to the hospital and I will find my son Noble Thomas to be revived. I arrive at the hospital and I find a wheelchair, asking my dad to rush me to my son, Noble.

We find the room where my mom, my pastor, my friend Kathy, Eugene, my dad and a nurse are all sitting around Noble. My mom hands me my baby, Noble, and I look at him. His eyes are shut and he is not moving. My whole body travails and shakes uncontrollably as I cry out the most guttural, deep shrieks I have ever heard escape my mouth. The shrieks echo throughout the entire hospital. I hold my baby and rock my body up and down, up and down, while holding Noble and shrieking, "no, no, no, not my baby, not my baby, no, no, no, not my baby, no God, not my baby, don't take my baby, no, no, no." This process continues for a long time, probably 45-minutes. My mom, sitting across from me, begins to cry and rock back and forth, back and forth, with me like there is a rhythm to the terrible grief that overtook us. And all of a sudden, I stop, hand my baby to my pastor and ask him to pray. My mind still could not register that Noble was dead. I fought between outright denial, shock and intense overwhelming grief that would overtake my entire body.

The thalamus in the brain acts like a relay station to pull in sensations. The thalamus can break down during trauma leading some people to lack a complete narrative like the one I just shared with you about Noble. Sometimes after trauma, a victim experiences only isolated sensory imprints like images, sounds and physical sensations accompanied by intense emotions of terror and helplessness.[3]

When the thalamus shuts down after an experience of trauma, the victim can also experience compromise in attention and concentration, with new learning becoming impossible after the experience. Some trauma victims completely dissociate from themselves during the overwhelming experience.[4] This leads to fragmented emotions, sounds, images and thoughts that are relived over and over again while the trauma remains unresolved. Often times, stress hormones keep circulating in the body, intense emotional responses are replayed and a defensive posture is developed.

Developing PTSD after trauma allows the floodgates of the senses to be wide open with no filter. In such a state, a person experiences sensory overload and cannot cope with life. Some people in a state of PTSD develop tunnel vision and hyper focus. Others shut themselves down while some trauma victims use drugs or alcohol in an attempt to cope.[5]

After my son died, I developed a hyper focus on my business and began to develop the videos for my program, Cancer Peace University. The hyper focus and tunnel vision on my business helped me to cope with a seemingly hopeless and tragic loss. I was able to find meaning in the ashes of loss through serving the needs of my clients with a life-threatening diagnosis. This helped me to find structure and regain my mental acuity.

There are many challenges when working with someone who has experienced trauma in childhood and/or trauma as an adult. People who have experienced trauma struggle to live fully and securely in the present. In order to transition into living fully in the present, the brain structure that stopped functioning when the person was overwhelmed with trauma needs to be reactivated. There are many potential areas of the brain that can become shut down because of trauma. In fact, the reflex of purpose in the brain can be damaged in trauma victims, which can lead them to become very disorganized and purposeless.[6] Humans thrive with purpose as it helps to organize our way through the world.

Pavlov was a researcher who is well known for his accidental experiment with his dogs in 1924. The river flooded in Pavlov's basement lab, which caused his dogs to become trapped. The dogs all survived but exhibited signs of intense trauma. In fact, weeks after the water receded, the dogs acted as if they were still in grave danger. A new internal equilibrium was found after the trauma, which caused the dogs to live hyper vigilant to threats and caused them to mistrust their environment. The trauma was complicated for the dogs because their physical impulse to run from the rising water was impeded as they were locked in cages. This led to inescapable shock and a complete breakdown in equilibrium. Because the dogs could do nothing to affect their fate as the water was rising, they were severely traumatized by their helplessness and inability to fight or flight. Instead of being able to fight or flight, the dogs were forced to freeze and become immobile.[7] Women in domestically violent relationships who feel that they have no way out can suffer from complicated cases of trauma and inescapable shock. Also, children abused by their parents are stuck in a catch-22: they need their parents for shelter, protection and food, and yet the people who are keeping them alive are also hurting them.

Further, Pavlov's research found that the pre-existing temperament of the dogs shaped how they responded to the stress after trauma. Dogs who were strong, excitatory, lively, calm or melancholic all responded very differently after their experience of inescapable shock.

Before the death of my son, I derived great meaning from helping my clients diagnosed with cancer address their diagnosis in a holistic manner. At 37 years of age, I also had developed a deep sense of emotional intelligence, conquered certain limitations and pain from my past and felt purposeful in the direction of my career. Thus, I believe that I moved through grieving as best as I could partly because I was in a good frame of emoting and had a very healthy sense of meaning in my life. Throwing myself further into my practice served to catapult my grieving and healing process.

Our sense of purpose involves movement and emotions. Emotions propel us into action and emotions are assets to organize a meaningful life around. The emotions of grief that I felt when three of my friends died of cancer propelled me into the cancer field. The death of my son brought me to the very center of my purpose in the cancer field. I dug even deeper into my purpose and the emotions of grief solidified my vision 100-fold. In my case, purpose was part of my healing. However, for others who experience a diminishing of their reflex of purpose, regaining purpose can become challenging after trauma. When someone experiences trauma that flattens the reflex of purpose in their brain, how do we help them to regain energy to engage with life in a meaningful way?

Shortly after our son, Noble Thomas, died, we struggled to remember anything and everything. My husband would go to a room in the house with an agenda and completely forget why he was in the room. I would run upstairs with a mission to find something and come downstairs empty-handed. I still remember one particular day when my husband and I discovered this forgetfulness pattern in our brains. We knew that it was connected to the trauma of Noble Thomas dying.

The brain has two main systems that are relevant for the mental processing of trauma: the amygdala and the medial prefrontal cortex. The emotional intensity of an event is processed through the amygdala. The context and meaning of an experience is processed and determined through the dorsolateral prefrontal cortex and the hippocampus. In fact, the dorsolateral prefrontal cortex tells us how our present experience relates to our past and how it may affect our future. When we know that our experience is finite and will come to an end, most experiences are tolerable.[8] However, when situations feel like they will last forever, the trauma remains unresolved and becomes intolerable.

After trauma, it is common to experience the breakdown of parts of the brain. The shut-down of parts of the brain can hinder someone's ability to process and resolve the trauma in a meaningful manner, but can affect anything from our ability to remember things to our ability to understand and process context and time. For example, if the dorsolateral prefrontal cortex shuts down, context and time are not understood and become skewed to the person surviving the trauma.

In some cases of trauma, the survivor may numb out completely with their mind going blank. In this case, the body does not register the trauma and the heart rate and blood pressure do not elevate. The survivor of trauma literally dissociates and leaves their body in response to the trauma. The medical term for this dissociation or blanking out is depersonalization.[9] People who dissociate during trauma shut down nearly every part of their brain to the point that they cannot think, feel, remember or make sense of the trauma. Talk therapy is completely useless for those who have survived trauma and dissociated during their experience.

In fact, after an experience of trauma, researchers have discovered a significant decrease of activity in an area of the brain called the Broca's area, which resides in the frontal lobe cortex. Broca's area is the speech center of the brain, which is often affected in a negative manner after a stroke. Without a functioning Broca's area, someone is unable to put thoughts or feelings into words.[10] Trauma is preverbal and often leaves people speechless. Broca's area is found to be completely offline whenever a flashback of trauma is triggered. Thus, trauma victims struggle to share stories of their experiences. Further, many victims of trauma find certain approaches to therapy to cause more harm than good as they are unable to verbalize what they have experienced.

In the days after losing Noble, my body trembled, convulsed and took on a life of its own when people would come to comfort my husband and I.

With community support, I was able to grieve, but the grief did not come out in words, as a cohesive story. Instead, family and friends would come to comfort me and I would collapse in their arms, shaking, screaming and wailing in uncontrollable travail. At the end of the intensely physical release of grief, I would feel a sense of relief, until the next wave of uncontrollable grief passed through my body.

Images of the past trauma will activate the right hemisphere while deactivating the left hemisphere of the brain. The two halves of the brain speak different languages with the right side being intuitive, emotional, visual, spatial and tactual. The left side of the brain is linguistic, sequential, and analytical and does all of the talking. The right side of the brain is the first to develop in the womb and carries nonverbal communication between mothers and infants.[11]

When an experience in the present reminds someone of a past trauma, the brain reacts as if the trauma is happening in present day reality.[12] This leads to emotional storms, blame and a general deactivation of the left hemisphere of the brain. There can be a lack of self-awareness when trauma is triggered because of diminished activity of the left hemisphere of the brain. Further, during trauma flashbacks, a person is unable to register long-term effects of actions, identify cause and effect or to create future plans.

In cases of unresolved trauma, stress hormones take much longer to return to baseline after stressful stimuli. In fact, stress hormones spike quickly and disproportionately in response to mildly stressful stimuli. When there is a constant elevation of stress hormones, memory and attention diminish while a person becomes more irritable and can develop sleep disorders.[13] After my son died, my husband and I could not sleep through the night and would find ourselves wide-awake at different times throughout the night. I remember one night waking up to my husband sobbing uncontrollably. Of course, this triggered me to start crying as waves of grief ran through my body. We also could not remember basic things and struggled to make plans. Our brains were compromised because of the constant elevation of stress hormones from unresolved trauma.

In some cases, people who experience trauma stay in a state of denial. The conscious mind continues on with life as if nothing ever happened, but the body registers the threat of the trauma and the stress response system remains on heightened alert. The mind can learn to ignore messages from the emotional brain, but the alarm of threat does not stop resounding in the body. When traumatized people are presented with images, sounds and thoughts that are related to their experiences, the amygdala reacts with alarm, even years later.[14] The amygdala then triggers a cascade of stress hormones, nerve impulses, blood pressure increase, heart rate increase and starvation of oxygen as the body prepares for fight or flight. The physical effects continue within the body until the trauma is resolved or the body develops a disorder or disease.

I will never forget my first session with Pam. Full of emotion, Pam, began sobbing as she shared the depth of her despair with me, "For the first time in my life, I am experiencing the joy of being a grandma to my first grandson. I have had a hard life and joy seemed to evade me for many years. My husband was married to his job and I had two little babies right in a row. After my second child, I developed Type I Diabetes and could hardly function. I remember days that I would take both babies in my arms like footballs and army crawl up the stairs because of the pain and fatigue in my body. When I found out that I was pregnant with our 3rd child, I just knew I couldn't survive another pregnancy. I had an abortion. I had Type I Diabetes and my husband was married to his job. I had two little babies at home who needed me; I had no choice. I had to have an abortion."

I let Pam release all of her pent-up emotions as she jumped from trauma to trauma in her life. She already had won my heart. Endeared to my new client, I learned more and more about her challenging past and felt much compassion for her. I also felt admiration for what she had been through and survived. Pam continued with her story that first day after I asked her, "Why do you think you have cancer?" Pam retorted, "I know exactly where this tumor is from, which is why I need to get it out of me. My birth mother is still haunting me to this day. Why won't she ever leave me alone?"

Tears streaming down her face, Pam tried to gather herself, but continued to lay all of her emotions on the table. "The best thing that happened to me as a child was when our neighbor came over to watch us and found bruises on the backs of our legs. It confirmed the worst of her suspicion, as I am sure they overheard yelling and crying in our apartment often. The neighbor called CPS and we were taken from our home immediately and put up for adoption. My adoptive parents adopted me and their home was slightly better than my birth parent's home in the sense that I had all that I needed and there was no physical abuse when we were younger. However, I was treated like the help and learned to clean and cook and do whatever my adoptive mother needed me to do."

The 90-minutes quickly passed in our first session and I knew that Pam was ready to address the deeper causes of her diagnosis. She was very self-aware and brave to bear all of her emotions to me in the first session. It was no wonder that after all of the childhood trauma that Pam endured that she would be diagnosed with ovarian cancer. How could anyone face such tragic depth of abandonment, neglect and abuse and not have physical manifestations of disease?

Over the process of the next 2 years, Pam became my most devoted client. Just when we addressed one emotional root, another one surfaced and she would discover the next emotional root to her diagnosis. I was shocked at what one life could endure. Despite the hurt she endured as a daughter, Pam was a wonderful, devoted mother to her two children. She undid the transgressions of her mothers by committing to be the best mother that she could be.

One day, she shared with me her deeper fears regarding going to doctors, "When I was very young, like 4 or 5 years old, my brother and I ran to an abandoned warehouse. We were alone and unsupervised a lot as children, so trips like this were nothing new. I remember finding an abandoned warehouse and trying to break into the door. As we went into the back of the warehouse, I fell through some wood to the basement of the building. When I landed, I fell on some glass and was bleeding profusely. I yelled to my brother to help me and he rushed to my rescue, finding a way to the basement. He ran me home to a horrified mother who rushed us to the hospital. The doctors treated me like nothing and didn't try to sooth or calm me as I was in a frantic state. They just treated me like business as usual and didn't listen to me as I screamed, "Stop, you are hurting me!" In fact, they did stiches on my face, but they didn't give me enough pain medication so I felt the entire thing as it happened. I never trusted doctors again after that day. I feel so much fear and panic arise in my chest when I see a doctor as a result of this experience."

Taking it all in, I tell her calmly, with much compassion, "Pam, let's try to redesign this memory together. What would you say to those doctors if you had been able to speak to them and they were able to listen to you?"

Pam took a deep breath and said, "I would have said, I'm a little girl. Do you have a daughter, a granddaughter or a niece who you love? I have a mother, a grandmother, grandfather and an aunt who all love me. Can you treat me like you would your own daughter? Can you show me love and listen to me? You hurt me so much when you didn't listen to me, when you didn't even try to calm me down. You ignored my cries and screams like I was nobody to you and not worth anything. I felt like trash, like nothing and my whole life I have been terrified of doctors because of you."

Pausing to get a tissue, Pam took a deep breath in and out. I waited. And then I said the following, "Can you try to forgive the doctors in the memory for what they did to you?"

Pam closed her eyes again and pursed her lips. "I can try. I choose to forgive you, I hated you for years, but today I choose to forgive you."

"Great, how does the memory feel now?" I asked her softly. Pam answered, "It feels less intense and chaotic. But I still feel so sad."

"Pam, can you release your sadness by saying, I release this sadness to God." I responded.

Pam replied, "Yes, I give this sadness to God."

I saw more tears streaming down her face as I said the following, "God, we invite you into this memory to speak, heal and restore Pam. Show Pam something that she doesn't know." We waited for a few moments.

A look of calm came over Pam's face as she opened her eyes and said, "It's gone now. The memory was swallowed up by a black hole. I can't even see it anymore. I feel free. Thank you."

Some of my clients can go through 2 years of trauma, releasing, remembering, forgiving and redesigning memories, like Pam did. Others only have a few small moments of pain and trauma still lingering in their system. Either way, the mind and body does not forget trauma and if it is not resolved fully, trauma will manifest one way or another.

Take some time to visit the companion workbook to process any past trauma that may be lingering for you. Cancer can be a wake-up call to take back your life and to allow parts of you that have been dead to come back alive again. Trauma is like a dead tooth that needs to be extracted for the body, mind and soul to flourish again. Let's remove your past traumas together in the companion workbook.

Section 3: Unraveling the Imprint of Trauma

Chapter 2: Mindfulness: Ending the Phantom Existence

After breaking my own heart and ending my relationship with Joe, I struggled to move forward and embrace life. In some ways, I traumatized myself because I had been so obsessive and possessive of the relationship. Over a period of several years, I trained my brain to believe that Joe was my husband and that there were no other options. This caused me to become exceedingly unhappy and disengaged with life. I slowly began to engage in new friendships that helped me cope with this major loss in my life.

Jonathon and I connected through mutual friends one night and I remember an instant connection as we both tended towards deep thinking and emoting that allowed us to sync and flow in conversation. I felt instantly mirrored, heard and attuned with my friend, Jonathon. He intuitively knew things about me that most people learned about me over time, "You are a safe place for people. People are drawn to you and can relax and open up all of their deepest pains and emotional traumas. You are full of empathy and love for people." I felt seen and understood by Jonathon. And I found a relational space where I could purge my deepest emotional pain connected to losing Joe.

I remember thinking to myself, "How can life continue without my relationship with Joe?" He was all that I knew for six years of my life. Joe helped to ease the emotional pain of life and helped me to feel known and loved in a unique way that no one else had previously. When I found Joe, I no longer felt alone and abandoned. I felt that I had someone who cared deeply about my emotional experience in life and would always be there for me in a depth that I had never experienced before.

However, after I became friends with Jonathon, I realized that there were other people that I could emotionally share life with and feel a similar support. Jonathon became one of my best friends and my greatest confidant in a deeply stressful time in my life.

In 1994, Stephen Porges, a researcher at The University of Maryland explained why a kind face or soothing voice can alter dramatically how we feel. Being seen and heard by important people in our lives can make us feel calm and safe. However, being ignored or dismissed can trigger rage and even mental collapse. Focused attunement with a mother type figure can shift us out of a fearful and disorganized state.[1]

Jonathon was my mother type figure (don't tell him that, I'm not sure he would be enamored by this). He became like an emotional doula to me and I was able to purge the deepest emotions in the loss of my relationship with Joe. I remember one specific instance when I was with Jonathon and I discovered a deep release of emotional pain after sharing my feelings: "I just don't understand. I remember when we found out that my dad and Joe had the same nickname in high school. My dad's nickname was Sid and so was Joe's! This felt so strange, yet I thought it was a sign that we were meant to be together. Another time, I was with Joe and his mother and she took off her beautiful gold bracelet that had a heart charm on it and put it on my wrist. She said softly to me, 'I will tell you more about this one day. But for now, you can keep it.' I took this as another sign that we were supposed to be together. It just doesn't make sense to me. I never felt as happy as I did when I was with Joe. But now, I feel a void every day in my heart. I feel alone, like there is nothing for me."

Crying, I felt like my words missed the depth of the tragedy that I felt in losing Joe. But when I looked across the couch at my friend Jonathon, I saw in his eyes that he understood me. He felt what I could not verbalize and he was holding it all for me in such a beautiful way. He sat, pondering what to say to comfort me. And then, in a way that only friends can do in a moment of emotional pain, he cracked a joke: "Joe will probably come to your wedding and confess his undying love for you in front of everyone, asking for the wedding to stop." Laughing with Jonathon at the absurdity of that image, I began to relax and feel supported in my deep emotional turmoil.

Our brains are built innately to help us function well in community. In 1994, Italian scientists identified specialized cells in the frontal cortex called mirror neurons.[2] Mirror neurons allow for a child to watch a parent, imitate them and learn how to engage socially with the world. Mirror neurons help us to register another person's internal experience.[3] Interestingly enough, children with autism have been discovered to not express mirror neuron activity in their brains.

Mirror neurons explain empathy, imitation, synchrony and the development of language. Mirror neurons pick up on another person's movement, emotional state and even intentions. Mirror neurons allow for syncing with another person in a relationship. When people are in sync with one another, they will sit or stand in a similar manner and their voices will take on the same rhythms.

Jonathon and I experienced the rare, but beautiful type of syncing in a relationship that happened instantaneously instead of over a period of time. We could be surrounded by other friends and focus intently on each other's thoughts, feelings and internal experience and be completely in tune with one another. My friendship with Jonathon has been quite literally one of the best friendships of my life that helped me to process the most painful relational losses of my life.

Traumatized people find themselves chronically out of sync with people around them for many reasons. When someone has experienced trauma, boundaries were crossed that caused the person to not feel seen, heard or mirrored. Their internal experience was not taken into consideration. Trauma victims need to reactivate the capacity to safely mirror and be mirrored by others and learn to not be overtaken by someone's depression or negativity. When boundaries are crossed, mirror neurons can be misappropriated and now the very thing that allows us to sync with others relationally can make us vulnerable to being overtaken by another person's internal experience.[4] Another person's negativity, anger or depression can become our own if we have not developed the right boundaries in relationships or if trauma allowed for boundaries to be crossed.

The vagus nerve is our social engagement system, which depends on nerves that start in our brain. The vagus nerve is known as the caretaking nerve and this nerve registers heartbreak and gut-wrenching feelings. The dorsal vagal complex (DVC) is activated if there is no way out of a traumatic experience and if strategies of social support and engagement in fight or flight have both failed.[5] Now, we freeze or collapse. The symptoms expressed after freezing or collapsing include: reduced metabolism, plummeting heart rate and difficulty breathing. Other symptoms of the DVC taking over the nervous system are symptoms of diarrhea, nausea and shallow breathing.

One of the major symptoms that continued for 1 year after I lost Noble Thomas was an inability to catch my breath. The day after Noble died, my heart rate kept plummeting and I couldn't breathe properly. In order to ensure that there wasn't physically anything wrong with my lungs, my doctors ordered a CT scan. The scan showed what I had already assumed; there was nothing physically wrong with my lungs. Rather, my attempts to enlist social help by having doctor's work to resuscitate Noble Thomas failed. Fighting for my baby's life failed. The death of my baby became unavoidable and I collapsed from grief. When the DVC takes over, a person can lose touch with themselves and their surroundings and become almost immobile.

A month prior to the 1-year anniversary of Noble's death, my husband and I went to a retreat center called Faith Lodge. Faith Lodge held group counseling support every weekend of the year for families needing to process the grief involved with losing children. We and 4 other families gathered to share our stories, grieve and process where we were at in the death of our child. Prior to going on the retreat, I created a video for Cancer Peace University. I watched the video and it sounded like I just ran a marathon prior to making the video. Up until that point, I didn't realize how tangible and apparent my inability to breathe was to the rest of the world as it was to myself. Now I had tangible proof of the trauma and grief that had settled into my lungs and hindered my breathing.

The weekend was very healing as we shared our experience with a group of parents who walked the same path as us and understood our grief. My husband and I were mirrored, heard and seen with empathy and love. We were able to share our son Noble's story with an audience who embraced the pain and vulnerability, and saw their own loss through our experience. My husband and I wrote encouraging letters to each couple in our retreat group and presented them to each couple with a blessing and a prayer of support. To be a part of other couple's healing from grief actually brought a deeper healing to my own experience. We left feeling renewed, like we had expressed a deeper place of our grief.

The following week, I redid the lecture that I had done the previous week. When I watched the video, I was astonished. My breath had completely normalized. I saw nothing of the breathing issues that were so apparent just the week previously. It felt like I had witnessed a complete and utter miracle. The trauma and grief dissipated from my lungs, and I was free to breathe again. I felt complete closure in that moment and knew that I had been given the gift of wholeness after a year of complete brokenness.

Trauma will increase the risk of misinterpreting whether a situation is dangerous or safe. Faulty alarms from trauma lead a person to either blow up or shut down. I still remember almost having a panic attack when my phone would ring months after Noble died. I believed that I would answer the phone only to find out that another person had died or was deathly ill. In the brain, a shift in Medial Prefrontal Cortex (MPFC) activity makes it harder to control emotions and impulses. The critical balance between the amygdala and the MPFC shifts when someone develops PTSD after trauma. The MPFC offers a larger view on the event, helps us to observe what is happening, predict what may happen and make a conscious choice.[6] In highly emotional states, when MPFC activity reduces, people leave their senses and can startle in response to a loud noise (like a cell phone), become enraged by small frustrations or freeze when someone touches them.[7]

Mindfulness is the ability to hover calmly and objectively over thoughts and emotions, taking our time to respond to relational interactions and experiences. The executive brain can organize, modulate and inhibit automatic reactions of the emotional brain. To manage emotions better, we can either regulate emotions from the top-down or the bottom-up. Top-down regulation involves strengthening the capacity of MPFC to monitor the body's sensations. Strategies include journaling, developing mindfulness and meditation. Bottom-up regulation includes recalibrating the autonomic nervous system by way of breathing exercises, movement, touch and massage.

Eventually, you need to revisit the trauma directly, but only after you feel safe and will not be re-traumatized by it. In order to feel safe in the body and become mindful, connecting to our body through movement can help to restore balance to the brain and activate more self-awareness. Limbic System Therapy is approaching traumatic stress by restoring proper balance between the emotional and rational brain.

Many times, those who have experienced trauma will be triggered by every day interactions and feel the emotional brain taking over. Trauma victims may actually feel like their mind and body become hijacked by situations that trigger trauma. Trauma victims report the following symptoms after being triggered: gut-wrenching sensations, anxiety, a racing heart, shallow breathing, heartbreak, defensiveness, rigidity, rage and collapse. The body can be triggered into hyper or hypo arousal and a person who has been traumatized can become reactive, disorganized, overtaken by rage, panic, numbness or experience intruding images in the mind.[8]

Neuroscientist Joseph LeDoux found that the only way we can access the emotional brain is through developing self-awareness. The part of the brain that is involved in self-awareness is the Medial-Prefrontal Cortex.[9] The only way that we can change how we feel is by becoming aware of our inner experience and learning to befriend what is going on inside of us.

I remember months after my friend, Sherry, died of breast cancer, I went to the YMCA to swim laps, as was my habit. My brain felt sluggish and I was not very motivated. I didn't feel like I was making much progress. I called my mentor on the way home from the YMCA to try to describe how I was feeling. I said that I felt unmotivated, sluggish, fatigued and had little joy in life anymore. My mentor simply listened and reflected back to me the following, "I think that you are depressed after the death of Sherry. You are grieving." In that moment, it all clicked. I understood how I was feeling and why.

When I was able to recognize the depression I was feeling as a normal phase of my grieving, I was able to move past that phase. Within a few days, I felt more like myself and found myself coming out of the depression. Our minds are meant to make meaning out of our feelings and experiences. When we can understand our feelings through self-awareness, we can release those feelings and move on with living.

Eighty percent of the fibers of the vagus nerve, the care-taking nerve, run from the body into the brain connecting the brain to internal organs.[10] We can train our arousal system by the way that we breathe, chant and move. Movement such as dance, Pilates, sports, massage, kickboxing and running can help reconnect the brain to the body and help to create more body awareness. This in turn reduces stress hormones in the body and alleviates some of the PTSD symptoms after trauma.

In college, I studied Spanish as one of my majors and had the opportunity to travel abroad in Spain. I traveled to Italy on a long weekend and toured an area where I stumbled upon an old monastery. Climbing up the hundreds of steps of this great historical sanctuary, I became aware of a faint rhythm being released from the open doors of the monastery. As I grew closer, the sounds captivated my mind and body and I remember feeling euphoric as I listened to the angelic Gregorian chants. It must have been the most intoxicating, beautiful sound that I had ever heard in my life.

The music was so soothing that I have no doubt in the power of music therapy when the sound and rhythm connects to the fractured human soul. Listening to music, as a therapy is one approach, while participating in the rhythm and music in dance, chorus, drumming and instruments with other people can dampen a stress response, wake up the Medial Prefrontal Cortex and lessen the symptoms of PTSD.[11] No wonder why I was drawn to Lindy Hop dance after the loss of my son, Noble Thomas. Dancing in rhythm with fellow human beings, I couldn't help but smile and laugh despite the heaviness and despair in my life from grieving. Dancing became an informal part of my therapy.

Developing body awareness through movement, athletics and dance puts us in touch with our inner world, helps us to notice subtle changes and helps to shift our perspective. Further, the practice of mindfulness helps us to take note of the transitory nature of our feelings. When we pay attention to our bodily sensations, we recognize that emotions ebb and flow. As we grow in mindfulness, we learn to recognize and release emotions while increasing our ability for self-management.

After trauma, some people become afraid of noticing their feelings. Emotions tend to flow in an unpredictable manner with a high level of intensity after trauma. Thus, many people become apprehensive of being hijacked by uncomfortable physical sensations that interrupt their ability to function in day-to-day life.

Because the speech center of the brain shuts down and the right hemisphere of the brain registers the trauma instead of the left hemisphere, talk therapy does not tend to help with trauma. In fact, talk therapy can make trauma worse in some cases. The rational brain simply cannot talk the emotional brain out of its own reality. After trauma, the soul, the body, the mind and the nervous system are different entities altogether. This is why most people will say after trauma, "I just don't feel like myself." **After a traumatic experience, energy is spent suppressing the inner chaos instead of spontaneously living life.**

Some people need to use a bottom-up approach in dealing with trauma by engaging their physiology first. Dance, rhythmic interactions, joining a choir or band, tossing a beach ball back and forth, bouncing on a Pilates ball, drumming or massage can all help the body to begin to engage again. This type of approach calms down the stress response system, helps the brain connect with the body again and wakes up areas of the brain that shut down during trauma. I remember feeling an urge to dance after the trauma of losing Noble. As I began to Lindy Hop dance on a regular basis, I found that it was the one place where I felt fully alive and joyful. My brain focused on the movement and the energy of the dance, while my stress response system transitioned out of high alert. In a way, I was communicating to my brain and my body that the trauma had ended and eventually, we were going to be okay and move forward with living.

Dancing and movement help to express emotions that many people cannot verbalize after surviving a major trauma. In fact, some people develop something called alexithymia as a result of trauma. Alexithymia is a condition where someone literally has no words for their feelings. Traumatized adults and children may be unable to discern what physical sensations in their bodies mean. This causes them to be out of touch with what they need and makes it very challenging to care for their own needs. People with alexithymia substitute action words for emotional language.

For example, if you asked someone with alexithymia how they would feel if they saw a car driving towards them, about to hit them, they would respond by saying something like, "How would I feel? I would jump out of the way."[12] Someone with alexithymia registers emotions as physical problems instead of signals that need their attention. When researchers showed people with alexithymia pictures of people's faces who were angry and distressed, they could not figure out what the people were feeling.[13]

How does alexithymia affect the physical body? Someone with alexithymia continually suppresses their emotions and is almost completely unable to express their emotions. The physiological response to suppressing emotions is for the body to be under stress. Thus, the blood pressure rises and the core body temperature decreases, which leads to damage to the mitochondria. Suppressing emotions has an impact on the body similar to exposure to physical toxins. Negative emotions that are suppressed will recycle continually in the body and cause damage to the mitochondria like any other physical toxin. When there is enough damage to the mitochondria within a cell, the cell will send a distress signal to the genome to cause the cell to become an immortal fermenter of glucose or a cancer cell.

Trauma victims cannot recover until they befriend physical sensations in their body. Physical self-awareness is the first step to recovery. This is another reason why dancing and other physical movement helps a trauma victim. Body awareness develops with rhythmic movements and physical engagement, which can develop a foundation of awareness that feeds into emotional awareness. Journaling can also help someone connect to thought patterns and physical sensations in their body. Individuals who lack emotional awareness can, with practice, connect their physical sensations to psychological events. In this manner, they can begin to reconnect with themselves.[14]

"Double Sorrow"

I remember the beginning stages of overwhelming emotions of grief gripping my body and my mind after Noble died. I was speaking to my mentor in an attempt to verbalize what I was experiencing shortly after Noble died. The term that felt the most descriptive and accurate to my experience was the term "double sorrow." I had gone through the painful, difficult process of pregnancy and instead of receiving a baby with joy: I was met with sorrow. As a result, I felt that the loss of my baby would define my life as a "double sorrow." I felt like a stranger to myself. Everything seemed to spiral out of control. I had to begin the slow and painful process of rebuilding my life after trauma.

Agency is the feeling of being in charge of your life. Agency begins with a process of introspection, which means to develop an awareness of our subtle sensory, body-based feelings. The greater level of self-awareness we can develop, the greater potential we possess to control our lives. In fact, knowing what we feel is the first step to knowing why we feel that way. **Mindfulness practice is simply the practice of observing what is happening inside of our body, mind and emotions.** Mindfulness practice is cornerstone to recovery from trauma.[15]

Thankfully, prior to the major trauma in my life, I had developed a fairly high level of emotional intelligence and could connect with the physical sensations in my body. I had years of practice of mindfulness and habits of meditation, journaling and prayer to undergird my grieving process. If the trauma of losing a child occurred prior to my development of a mindfulness practice, I am unsure how I would have been able to navigate the landmines involved in grieving and processing a major trauma. I would have possibly gotten stuck in complicated grief with an overall recovery taking longer. Thankfully, it took about 1 year for me to recover and regain my sense of agency after Noble died. But that year was marked with uncertainty, emotional ups and downs and a bit of chaos, as my internal world was shook to the core.

I relied on social support and community that was well established as my body went into survival mode and had heightened hyper vigilance to new relationships. In fact, researchers discovered that people with PTSD could not activate their Frontal Lobe. As a result, they could not be curious about a stranger. Our Prefrontal Cortex helps to assess a person coming towards us and mirror neurons interpret the intentions of that person. Researchers found that people with PTSD startled in response to a stranger while engaging in self-protective behaviors. There was no activation of any part of the brain involved in social engagement; instead, the person suffering from PTSD went into survival mode.[16] I had a friend move home to Minnesota for a period of time after I had intense PTSD and I could not connect or engage in this past relationship because of the intense shut down of my brain after trauma.

Researchers discovered that some people experience the loss of self after trauma. This is known as depersonalization. Paul Schilder, a German psychoanalyst found that the depersonalized individual experiences the world in a dream-like state. In fact, objects appear diminished in size and sounds come from a distance. Emotions are altered and the person in a depersonalized state experiences no pain or pleasure. They have become complete strangers to themselves and live a phantom existence.[17]

Depersonalization and alexithymia are the most extreme types of reactions to trauma and can be the most challenging to shift. The release and resolve of trauma begins and ends with the willingness and motivation of the individual trapped in their past experience of trauma. **Some trauma victims choose, unfortunately, to live trapped in past trauma instead of slowly moving towards rebuilding their lives.** In this case, self-regulation and agency are not developed, but external regulation becomes the norm. Medications, drugs, alcohol, compulsive compliance or people pleasing (to avoid uncomfortable emotions and conflict) and constant reassurance are needed to function. Some trauma victims develop extreme eating disorders in an attempt to externally regulate control while their internal world is thrust into absolute chaos with no resolve.

Traumatized people who have not resolved past traumas feel unsafe in their bodies while they are bombarded by internal warnings. In an attempt to control their lives, trauma victims ignore gut feelings and numb their awareness by learning to hide from themselves. While ignoring or distorting body's messages, a trauma victim becomes unable to detect what is dangerous between what is nourishing. Further, the stress of unresolved trauma impacts the biochemistry of the body in a myriad of ways. Migraine headaches and asthma attacks, chronic back and neck pain, fibromyalgia, digestive problems and chronic fatigue can all develop as somatic symptoms with no clear physical basis.[18]

Now, let's look at the exercises and questions in your companion journal to learn the practice of mindfulness and to begin the steps necessary to rebuild your life after trauma. Even if you are living with the effects of childhood trauma, it's never too late to open up to heal and resolve the effects of trauma on your physiology.

Section 3: Unraveling the Imprint of Trauma

Chapter 3: Become a Curious Observer of Your Internal World & Own Your Emotional Brain

The sound of a basketball bouncing up and down, up and down, up and down, pierced my overwhelming thoughts and emotions. A needed distraction, my eye gaze met the eyes of the basketball player, a petite child with frosted over eyes, grimaced his face and shot the ball. It hit the backboard like a ton of bricks and bounced over to me. Grabbing the ball, I called out to him, "Hey, come over here, I want to know your name."

He reluctantly walked over to me and said quietly, "My name is Anthony Jr., but people call me Junior." He stared at me with an empty look in his eyes, hiding any emotion and seeming to try to block any personal connection with me.

"So, what's your story?" I tried to ask casual to see what he had to say to me.

"Not much to my story. My dad drank a bottle of gin like he does, beat up my mom and now we are here, stuck at this hell-hole with all kinds of a-holes."

Junior spoke with aggression and overt resentment towards the shelter.

Considering his words, my mind raced to find the right response to help alleviate his struggle. Intuitively, I knew there was nothing I could do to rescue Anthony Jr. from his life full of pain. I also knew that I couldn't promise to even be there for him tomorrow, much less in the future. Admittedly, I had gone to the shelter in hopes of adding more community service to my growing resume as I applied to college after college, hoping to be accepted into some Ivy League Universities. It seemed so petty now as I looked at the shattered lives that came from the most horrific home environments one could conceive. I shouldn't even be here right now, I thought to myself. I felt a slight sense of shame as I realized my pride and selfishness motivating me to come to the shelter. I couldn't relate to the struggles of the children and moms who came to the shelter to flee their abusers. I also felt at a complete loss as to how I could add any value to their lives.

I was a teenager from a privileged upbringing and had never known anyone in poverty, abuse or any sort of situation that these mothers and children faced day in and day out. In that moment, I knew that my community service effort was a failed attempt and I couldn't even conceive of adding it to my list of achievements. However, that experience imprinted something deep upon my soul that I would later realize. It started with a question. How does someone help in situations of severe trauma and abuse? In my near future, I would search to gain the wisdom and knowledge to be in a position to help in these situations.

Just as Junior had done effortlessly, trauma victims often shut down parts of their brain simply to survive. In an attempt to shut down terrifying sensations from trauma, victims often shut down the area of the brain that allows for self-awareness. As a result, their relationship to their inner reality becomes impaired. This leads to a loss of purpose and direction in addition to a lack of self-awareness, while protecting the trauma victim from emotional pain.

Dr. Lanius performed a study to understand exactly how trauma affects sensory self-awareness. In the study, he compared Canadians with no history of abuse to people with a history of child abuse.[1] Through brain scans, Lanius found that the Default State Network or DSN was activated in those with no history of child abuse and mainly shut down in those with a history of abuse. The DSN is paramount to our ability to develop a sense of self. More specifically, the study found that the Medial Prefrontal Cortex, Insula, Anterior Cingulate and Parietal Cortex were active for those with no history of abuse and inactive in the brains of those with a history of abuse. The Insula relays messages from the Viscera to emotional centers in the brain while the Parietal Cortex integrates sensory information. The Anterior Cingulate coordinates emotions and thinking. The Posterior Cingulate acts as an internal GPS to give us a sense of where we are located in the world. In addition, the

Posterior Cingulate was the only part of self-awareness in the brain to be active in both those with no history of abuse and those with a history of abuse.

Part of the goal in working with people with a history of trauma and abuse is to find ways to reactivate the self-sensing system. The first step in reactivating self-awareness is to develop emotional intelligence and self-awareness in present day reality. If you cannot tolerate your feelings now, opening up the past can re-traumatize you.[2] If you have unresolved trauma from your past, you may need to revisit the first section of this book to solidify your emotional intelligence and self-awareness in the present before addressing past traumas.

Mindfulness can be developed as we start with the basics of journaling, meditation, body awareness, organizing our thoughts and pinpointing our emotions and bodily sensations. Mindfulness has been shown to impact positively symptoms of depression, chronic pain, immune impairment, high blood pressure and elevated cortisol levels.[3] Mindfulness also activates brain regions involved in emotional regulation, which leads to changes in brain regions involved in body awareness and fear.[4] When we find balance between our rational and emotional brain, we can develop self-mastery; learning to control our thoughts and emotions instead of feeling hijacked by our soul realm when we are triggered by the past.

Change begins when we learn to own our emotional brain. We can learn to observe and tolerate physical sensations in our body, while we develop the ability to verbalize and express a wide-range of emotions. Start now by committing yourself to be a curious observer of your internal world. Decide to stop suppressing bodily sensations and emotions. If you have spent most of your life trying to squash emotional awareness, this will be a challenge at first. Calming techniques such as breathing exercises can help. Breathe deeply in and out 6 times, following the sensations of your breath into your body. Now, keep your mind alive and engaged in this process. Allow your body to feel the feelings you suppress and normally dread. Stand back and observe yourself in an open and curious manner.

Childhood trauma is radically different than traumatic stress in fully formed adults. Thus, the trauma that Junior was experiencing was going to require more to overcome than for his mother, unless she also had trauma as a child instead of just traumatic stress as an adult. Women with an early history of abuse and neglect are 7 times more likely to be raped as an adult.[5] Further, children who witness their mothers being assaulted by their partners have a higher chance of being in an abusive relationship as an adult.

The actions, words and beliefs of our parents shape the way that we perceive reality. From the womb to seven years of age, we develop our core belief system in the subconscious mind. During childhood, we make conclusions about our reality, interpreting and translating our experiences into a cohesive belief system. Our core belief system undergirds our worldview and helps us to engage the world around us. Our subconscious mind stores our core belief system in the form of memories that carry the conclusions that we came to during childhood experiences. In a split second, our subconscious mind accesses our belief system in our memories to interpret the world around us and to aid in our interactions and decisions in life. Trauma during childhood has a broader impact on someone's life primarily because of how it can skew the core belief system while it is being formed. Our interactions with our caregivers convey what is safe and what is dangerous, whom we can depend upon and what we need to do in order to have our needs met. Thus, trauma can skew the vantage point in which we interact with others, the spiritual world and ourselves.

If someone is held down, trapped or prevented from taking effective action during trauma, they are at risk for developing PTSD at the same time that the body continues in a state of fight or flight. During war, a car accident, domestic violence, rape or childhood abuse, the brain keeps secreting stress chemicals to induce a proactive response long after the trauma is over.[6] Those in a domestically violent relationship often times are threatened and manipulated; as a result, they don't feel free to act and leave the relationship. They may be emotionally and financially dependent on their abusive partner or have children with their abuser. In addition, they may receive threats that hinder their ability to make a clear action to find safety.

Researchers studying trauma have discovered that many trauma victims secrete stress hormones long after the actual danger has passed.[7] In a study on "inescapable shock," Maier & Seligman studied the impact of trauma on dogs that were shocked while being locked in cages compared to a control group. The control group was not shocked in the 1st phase. In the 2nd phase of the study, the cage doors were opened so the dogs could escape if they so desired. However, the dogs that were locked in the cages when they were shocked the first time responded by staying in the cages and not running away the second time that they were shocked. Thus, the researchers discovered the concept of learned helplessness from an experience of inescapable shock. The dogs that were not able to respond to their instinct to flee during the trauma of being shocked in the 1st phase of the study, learned to become frozen or helpless in a future situation of trauma. In order for the dogs to leave the cages after this learned helplessness, the researchers had to draw the dogs out of the cages.[8]

Trauma involving cases of war, car accidents where a person becomes trapped, a domestically violent relationship where someone is hindered from leaving or getting help, rape and childhood incest or abuse, are such cases of inescapable shock that can cause a person to develop learned helplessness. Just like the dogs were drawn out of the cages to learn how to escape and how to become proactive again, can victims of trauma who learn helplessness be physically taught to escape a threatening situation?

Community and social support are part of the solution to regain agency after trauma. We respond with 3 different physiological states when we feel threatened. First of all, we seek social engagement and call for support when we feel threatened. If no one comes, we operate out of fight or flight mode and either fight our way out or run away to safety. If we cannot get away or we are trapped, we will freeze or collapse.[9]

Social support provides powerful protection against becoming overwhelmed by stress and trauma. Social relationships can help to ground and shift us into a healing process after trauma. This is another reason why childhood abuse and neglect is so harmful. It literally sabotages a person's ability to trust social support and can lead to lifelong habits of social anxiety and isolation. When a primary caregiver abuses and neglects their child, they betray the trust of their child who is supposed to experience their primary caregiver as a safe haven. A huge internal conflict develops between the child's loyalty to the family of origin and escape from the pain of the abuse. When children are asked to disown powerfully negative experiences that they have survived in order to remain loyal to their caregivers, they unintentionally create mistrust, inhibition of curiosity, distrust of their own emotions and a tendency to feel like they are living in an alternate universe.[10] Chronic emotional abuse and neglect in childhood can be just as damaging as physical and sexual abuse.[11]

There are several ways in which childhood trauma can be quenched in the moment of the trauma: 1. If the child is able to take an active role and flee from their perpetrator to safety, the imprint of trauma will be lessened. 2. If parents are able to give cues, remain loving and explain what happened to them, while reestablishing the fact that home is safe, the impact of trauma will also be lessened. 3. If a child is able to reach safety and their stress response system calms down, the impact of trauma will also be diminished. If we escape danger, we can regain our senses. However, if the brain's alarm system is triggered and there is no escape, a child can dissociate or suffer PTSD and collapse or freeze as a result.

Research has found that those with a history of childhood sexual and physical abuse have a higher risk of repeated suicide attempts and self-cutting.[12] After 3 years of therapy, 2/3 of people with a history of suicidal tendencies and self-destructive behavior improved considerably. Patients, however, who did not improve, had no memories of feeling safe with anyone during their childhood. If someone carries a memory and feeling of safety with just one person, the bond and feeling of safety can be reactivated with another adult and trauma can be addressed more readily. However, if someone lacks a deep memory of feeling loved and safe, the receptors in the brain that respond to human kindness can fail to develop.[13]

Adults who survived child abuse tend to experience the following symptoms later in life: trouble concentrating, complaints of being on edge, self-loathing, trouble negotiating intimate relationships, veering from indiscriminate high-risk unsatisfying sexual involvement to total sexual shutdown, large gaps in memories, self-destructive behaviors and a whole host of medical problems. The Adverse Childhood Experiences or ACE study discovered the impact of childhood trauma later in life. Felitti and Anda studied 17,421 white, middle-class, middle-aged, well-educated and financially secure control participants and found that only 1/3 of the respondents had no adverse childhood experiences.[14] Some of the topics explored in the study-included physical and sexual abuse, emotional and physical neglect and mentally ill, addicted or incarcerated caregivers. One in ten participants said, "Yes" to the following question: Did a parent or other adult in the house swear at you, insult you or put you down often? One in four participants said, "Yes" to the following question: Did one of your parents push, grab, slap or throw something at you often? Finally, to the question: Did someone 5 years older than you touch your body in a sexual way, 28% of women and 16% of men responded, "Yes."

The ACE study demonstrated that adverse experiences were interrelated with children tending to experience more than one negative experience in childhood. For example, of the two-thirds of respondents who reported adverse experiences in childhood, 87% scored 2 or more adverse experiences and 16.7% scored 4 or more adverse experiences. Half of those with ACE scores of 4 or higher had learning or behavioral problems in school whereas those with a score of 0, only 3% had problems in school. In adulthood, higher ACE scores were found to correlate with increased workplace absence, financial problems and lower lifetime income as an adult.

In addition, higher ACE scores increased the risk of chronic depression in adulthood. Those with an ACE score of 4 or higher, 66% of women and 35% of men developed chronic depression. In comparison, those with an ACE score of 0, only 12% experienced chronic depression. Research shows that depressed patients without prior histories of abuse or neglect tend to respond better to antidepressants than patients with those backgrounds.[15] Here are a few more statistics discovered in the ACE study:

- When comparing the odds of suicide attempts between an ACE score of 0 and an ACE score of 6, researchers found a 5,000% increased risk of suicide attempts in adulthood.
- Those who received an ACE score of 4 compared to an ACE score of 0 were 7 times more likely to become an alcoholic as an adult.
- When examining the risk of IV drug use, researchers found that there was a 4,600% increased risk of IV drug use for someone who scored an ACE of 6 compared to someone with an ACE score of 0.
- Those who received an ACE score of 4 or more adverse experiences had an increased likelihood of experiencing rape as an adult. In fact, 33% of

those with a score of 4 or more were raped as an adult compared to only 5% with an ACE score of 0.

- For boys who witnessed domestic violence in their homes during childhood, researchers found a 7-fold increased risk of abuse occurring in their own relationships.[16]

- Researchers also found a correlation between ACE scores and physical health. For example, those with an ACE score of 6 or higher had a 15% increased risk of experiencing one of the 10 leading causes of death in America, including, chronic obstructive pulmonary disease, ischemic heart disease and liver disease. Further, they were twice as likely to develop cancer and 4 times as likely to develop emphysema.

- Researchers also discovered that those with higher ACE scores tend to engage in high-risk behaviors such as smoking, multiple sexual partners resulting in unintended pregnancies and STDs and unhealthy lifestyle and eating choices leading to obesity.

- Another unintended discovery of the ACE study was the link of obesity to those who experienced rape and incest as a child. Felitti interviewed a participant who was sexually abused as a child and found the trauma victim stating, "Overweight is overlooked and that's the way I need to be."[17]

Trauma in childhood has a larger imprint on the physiology and psychology of a person than trauma in adulthood. First of all, the brain is not fully formed in childhood and the developing brain will change its development based upon trauma. Secondly, a child that survives trauma will make conclusions about the world based upon this horrific experience. These conclusions are stored in the subconscious mind and build the foundational worldview of a person. As an adult, they will view the world through the lens of that trauma. Many emotional patterns, thought patterns and behaviors will stem from the maladaptive core beliefs created after the experience of childhood trauma.

When Pauline first became my client, she shared with me that she didn't know how much progress we would make on the emotional side because she had been in therapy for most of her life. Well aware of the childhood trauma that imprinted pain and maladaptive core beliefs into her soul, Pauline was very transparent and willing to do the deeper work that correlated to her cancer diagnosis. She shared the painful memories with diligence and one memory that she shared with me was the following: "When I was still very young, like 8 years old, my adoptive father would come into my bedroom every night and sexually abuse me. I was confused, hurt and ashamed. I didn't know what to do, so I stayed quiet and didn't say anything to my mom or to my dad. About one year after he had started coming to my room at night, I told him firmly, 'This is the last night that you will come to my room.' After I asserted myself in this manner, he didn't come again.

That experience just added to the shame of being adopted and not knowing my real parents. My adoptive parents showed love and care to me in certain respects, but I was treated differently than my siblings. I could tell that I was not the favorite and that my adoptive parents felt like they were doing me a favor." Pauline took a sharp breath in as she reflected on this deeply painful experience. Therapist after therapist, she shared this story in the hopes of finding freedom from the shame and secrecy that colored her upbringing.

In that tender, delicate moment, I paused, not wanting to say the wrong thing or cause further pain. I gently asked Pauline, "Would you be ready to redesign this memory?" Pauline thought for a moment and then responded, "Yes, let's see if we can undo this terrible experience in my life." Asking for divine intervention in my head, I dove into the memory with Pauline, "Walk through the memory with me stage by stage and explain how you are feeling in different parts of the memory and where the most pain is held."

Pauline closed her eyes and traced the memory again, "I'm lying in my bed and I see light coming underneath my bedroom door. I am anxious, waiting, hoping that he doesn't come tonight. I watch the door, full of fear and anxiety. I can't breathe. I hear footsteps. The door opens slowly and I see my dad's looming figure looking at me. I keep my eyes shut and try to pretend to be asleep. Maybe he will go away. Instead, he closes the door behind himself and comes to my bed. He gently eases himself into my bed. I am terrified. I don't want him to come near me. I don't understand what he is doing, but I know intuitively that it is wrong. I hold my breath as his large body presses against mine. I smell a foul smell coming from his mouth and to this day I can't stand the smell of gin. Finally, it's over and he leaves my room. I toss and turn in bed all night, as I cannot sleep. Peace and sleep evade me. I feel uncovered, shameful and unprotected. I feel marred too, like I lost my childhood innocence. I notice myself pulling inwardly at school and around other people like if I were to open my mouth and talk, I would say the wrong thing and all of us would end up in jail." Pauline stops, sobbing again. She struggles to say, "How much can one person endure? I wonder why I had to go through such deep pain and sorrow? And now this, cancer."

My heart heavy, I want to do all that I can do to ease the emotional pain of my client. Pauline was one of those clients who had become more than a professional exchange. She had become like family to me. "I'm going to ask you to do something that might be hard for you, but let's see if you can do this. Imagine your dad was the perfect dad, the dad who listened to everything you had to say, can you share with him how you felt in this memory?"

Pauline paused, "OK, I will try." Gathering herself and wiping the tears from her face, Pauline said softly, "I see myself sitting at the end of the bed, waiting for him to come. This time I'm not going to let it happen. When the door opens, my dad is surprised to see me up and not in bed. I look at him square in the eyes, 'Dad, I don't want you to come to my room anymore at night. I am scared. I can't breathe right when you come. I feel ashamed and scared. I feel hurt and alone. I don't want you to touch me in that way anymore. I just want you to be my dad and protect me like a dad should. I need you to be a dad and to realize that you are hurting me more than anyone ever has. Can you see what you are doing is wrong?" Pauline cried and shuddered as the question lingered in the air.

Gently, I invited Pauline deeper, "Can you go into the memory as an adult and give your little self a hug?" Pauline nodded her head yes as she said, "I see myself walking into the room as my dad disappears and my little self looks away, shy and uncertain. I come up to her and say, 'Do you know whom I am?' She looks up at me and nods her head, "No." I squat down on my knees and look her square in the eyes, 'I am you. I am all grown up, 50 years later. I want you to know that you are going to be okay. You meet a wonderful man and get married. Your husband takes care of you and is so steady and gentle. You have 2 beautiful children. And somehow, you are a good mother. You love your children and find joy in being a mom. You also become a grandmother to 2 amazing grandchildren. You find joy in life. I want you to know that even though your life is hard right now, you are going to make it and it's going to be okay. You will heal and you will find the right people to love you. Can I give you a hug?' Pauline hugs her little self." Next, I heard Pauline sighing a sigh of relief.

"How does that feel?" I softly asked Pauline. Wiping away her tears, she responded, "Good, that feels good."

I pressed a little further, "Do you think that you can forgive your dad for what he did and forgive your mom for not knowing and not protecting you?" Pauline nodded her head and said, "Dad, what you did was wrong. But I choose to forgive you because I need peace and so do you. Mom, I choose to forgive you for not protecting me from dad and for not intervening in his drinking habit."

Curious, I asked Pauline, "How does the memory feel now?" Pauline closed her eyes and paused, "It feels better, more distant, lighter. But I still feel sad and alone." I responded, "I'm glad that it feels better. That is good progress. Now, I'm going to invite God into the memory with you. God, can you come into the memory and show Pauline what she needs to know?"

We waited. A few moments passed until Pauline opened her eyes and said to me, "It is done. I can't see the memory anymore and I feel peace. Thank you." We both sighed deeply in relief and gratitude for the freedom and peace that Pauline found in that memory.

A study performed in 1975 followed at-risk children from 130 families for 30 years, starting when the child was 3 months old.[18] Researchers discovered several parent-child dynamics to be problematic to behavior, learning and coping skills long-term. First of all, insensitive, pushy and intrusive parental behaviors at 6 months of age predicted hyperactivity and attention problems in kindergarten and beyond.[19]

Children who were regularly pushed over the edge into over arousal and disorganization did not develop proper attunement of inhibitory and excitatory brain systems. These children could lose control if something upsetting happened. On the other hand, children who received consistent caregiving became well-regulated kids. Erratic caregiving, however, produced kids who were chronically physiologically aroused.

Children of unpredictable parents clamored for attention and became intensely frustrated with small challenges. Further, they were chronically anxious, nervous and non-adventurous as a result of the unpredictability. In addition, early parental neglect and harsh treatment led to behavioral problems in school, troubles with peers and lack of empathy for the distress of others.[20] The most important predictor of how well the participants coped with life's disappointments was the level of security established with primary caregiving during the first 2 years of life. Interestingly enough, resilience in adulthood could be predicted based upon the degree mothers viewed their 2-year-old as loveable.[21]

The last study that we will look at is a study done in 1986 on sexual abuse and female development.[22] Researchers examined 84 girls with a history of sexual abuse compared to a control group of 82 girls with the same age, race, class and family background. These girls were followed from 11 years of age for 20 years to discover how childhood sexual abuse affected the victims in adulthood. The sexually abused girls demonstrated many and varied negative outcomes including cognitive deficits, depression, dissociative symptoms, troubled sexual development, high rates of obesity and habits of self-mutilation. As the abused girls developed, more of them than the control group dropped out of high school, experienced illnesses, had abnormalities in their stress response system, experienced early onset puberty and were diagnosed with a psychiatric illness.

During the study, researchers interviewed the young girls on an annual basis. The trauma victims and control group participants were both asked to talk about the worst thing that happened to them the previous year. The non-abused girls displayed signs of distress, while the abused girls shut down and became numb. The tests measuring cortisol levels actually decreased as the abused girls explained their most stressful event instead of increasing as it did for the non-abused girls. The researchers concluded that over time, the body adjusts to the chronic stress of trauma and numbing starts to occur. In this situation, teachers, friends and others are not likely to notice that the girl suffering from abuse is upset because her body has developed a survival method of freezing and numbing emotions instead of expressing them readily. An abused girl no longer reacts to distress as she should and becomes detached to her emotional and internal experience in an effort to survive the chronic exposure to trauma.

Abused girls rarely had close friends during teenage years, but in adolescence experienced chaotic, traumatizing contact with boys their age. Non-abused girls had several friends with girls and 1 guy friend throughout the adolescence stage. Their contact with boys would gradually increase over time. Abused girls cannot trust and have a different development pathway. They tend to not socialize or have close friends, hate themselves, overreact or numb themselves in relational interactions, and became sexually mature 1.5 years faster than the non-abused girls. According to the conclusion of the study, the abused girls could not articulate what they wanted, needed, nor could they think about how to protect themselves.

One study discovered abnormalities in the immune system response for those who experienced the trauma of incest as a child.[23] Researchers discovered that the proportion of those immune cells ready to attack is larger than normal for those with a history of incest. The immune system is found to be oversensitive to threat, ready to attack and can more easily attack self-tissue leading to autoimmune conditions. Incest victim's bodies literally have trouble knowing the difference between danger and safety.

For 1 year after the death of my son, I navigated many symptoms associated with trauma. Thankfully, in my case, I was able to find closure and healing throughout the process of grieving. However, I remember not being able to breathe for almost 1 full year. Until one day, miraculously, my breath came back to me. I remember not having an appetite and literally not eating for the majority of a year. My sleep was disturbed as I wrestled through the grief and reality of the trauma of losing my son.

When people relive trauma, nothing makes sense, they bounce between paralyzing fear or blind rage, food loses pleasure, sleep is disturbed and a desperation to escape intense bodily sensations through freezing or dissociation can occur.[24] Researchers discovered that after trauma, the Brodmann's area 19 in the brain relives the traumatic experience as though it was still occurring. Under normal conditions, the Brodmann's area 19 registers images of what has occurred and diffuses those images to other brain areas, which in turn interpret the meaning of what was experienced. However, the brain operates in a completely different manner in the aftermath of trauma.

The trauma continues to invade daily life when it remains active in the Brodmann's area 19. Sensory input through the eyes, nose, ears and skin converge in the thalamus where it is then sent to the amygdala in the limbic, unconscious part of the brain. The amygdala identifies information that is key to our survival and receives feedback from the hippocampus which compares new input to past experiences. Trauma is so different from past experiences that many times the brain lacks the capacity to process and integrate the experience with past experiences. In this case, the amygdala continues to sense a threat long after the trauma has occurred.

When the amygdala senses a threat, it sends a message to the hypothalamus and brain stem to act.

The hypothalamus and brain stem in turn recruits the stress response system and the autonomic nervous system to trigger sympathetic dominance. In a state of sympathetic dominance, the body releases cortisol, adrenaline and noradrenaline in order to increase the heart rate and blood pressure to prepare the body to run away or fight back. One of the greatest challenges after trauma is to reset physiology so that survival mechanisms stop working against the trauma victim. The goal is to help people with a history of trauma to reconnect to their body and mind in a way that allows their traumatic memories to be integrated as experiences from the past instead of the body living in a state of unresolved trauma where threat to survival is constantly perceived.

You cannot fully recover from trauma if you don't feel safe in your own body. Body-based treatments can help disrupt the physiological changes that occur in the aftermath of trauma to help calm down the stress response system. Further, body-based treatments help the person recovering from trauma to learn to feel safe and in charge of their own body. The most natural way to calm down distress is to be touched, hugged or rocked. This can help with excessive arousal and makes a person feel intact, safe and protected. A great body-based therapy to recover from trauma is seeking therapeutic massage and craniosacral therapy. After trauma, the body is physically restricted and emotions from the trauma are bound up inside the body. When physical tensions are released, emotions can be released as well.

The story of trauma can be in the backseat while a person explores physical sensations and discovers the imprint of trauma on their physiology. Other body-based therapies to explore include sensorimotor psychotherapy[25] and somatic experiencing.[26] Emotions can overwhelm a trauma survivor when they try to face the trauma head on; thus, using an approach of pendulation can be helpful. This approach swings in and out of the trauma, accessing sensations and emotions, while moving in and out of those feelings with sensitivity to avoid aggressive exposure to the memory.

Once a trauma victim can tolerate the physical sensations of their past experiences, they can begin to discover physical impulses like hitting, pushing, running and body movements such as twisting, turning and backing away that may have arisen during the trauma but were suppressed. Amplifying these movements can bring incomplete trauma-related action tendencies to a completion and can help to resolve the trauma. Treatments can include kickboxing, self-defense classes and running. When trauma victims can physically experience what it would have felt like to fight back or run away, they can relax, smile and feel a sense of completion.[27] The self-defense treatment approach can teach women or men to recondition the freeze response by learning to transform fear into positive fighting energy.

Traumatized people recover best in the context of relationships with family, loved ones or an alternative community approach like AA meetings or religious meetings. The role of relationships in healing from trauma cannot be discounted; however, not everyone is ready to start relating and sharing their deepest feelings. People who have a struggle to trust and open up in relationships may benefit from body-based treatments first. Once a person feels safe in their body, they may feel more able to communicate and relate in a healing environment with individuals or a community. Relationships can help people find freedom from the shame of their past actions or past traumatic incidents and allow them to move forward into healthy, intimate relationships.

Now it is time to explore your own experience with trauma in the companion workbook to this book, *Braving The Storm: In Pursuit of a Profound, Internal Transformation.* Open your companion workbook now to begin engaging with the questions and exercises relevant to the material in this chapter.

Section 3: Unraveling the Imprint of Trauma

Chapter 4: Reversing the Amnesia of Trauma to Fully Integrate Your Brain

"It's kind of hard growing up without a mom or a dad," Michael's voice cracked as he began to breakdown in tears. He struggled to find language to describe the depth of his broken, traumatic upbringing, but the emotion behind his words revealed much more than words ever could. The empathy in the room was palpable, as everyone seemed to take a breath in at the same time, feeling the depth of Michael's story. Overwhelmed at the response of the audience, Michael could hardly finish his story, while many of us were at a complete loss. I struggled to contain my emotions and began to sob in my seat with a deep sense of compassion for Michael and his broken childhood.

Everything stopped for several moments as Michael tried to collect himself before continuing. It was the first time that I had seen Michael become emotional in the span of knowing him for several years. He was always the first student to arrive at the high school in Cape Town and the last to leave. He took such pride in attending high school. I had volunteered at this particular high school that provided at-risk youth another chance at graduating, when they had lost other opportunities. Most of the students in the school came from a traumatic upbringing and for one reason or another never graduated from high school. Many had become involved in drug use, violence or gang activity and ended up dropping out or getting kicked out of high school. This particular school in Cape Town was their last chance to receive their high school diploma.

Michael was a model student, very respectful and well liked by teachers and students. From his smiling face and friendly disposition, you would have never known the depth of trauma that he had endured in his short life. In order to provide for the family, his mother would prostitute herself. His father was in jail and not available to be a real father and role model. Many times, his mother would use the money she earned to buy drugs and alcohol to numb the pain and shame of the reality of her life.

Michael basically raised himself and took the opportunity at the high school for at-risk youth very seriously. He was the model student and knew that this opportunity to excel and move beyond his parents' struggle with poverty, drugs and incarceration would possibly be his last. He graduated top of his class, but I'm unsure if the deep scars of his traumatic past had been sufficiently addressed. In all of my years as a counselor, I had never encountered such depth of trauma and emotional pain in the students at this particular high school. Talk therapy was useless, as the students could not find words to explain their past nor connect with any understanding to their emotional and relational experiences.

The majority of the students suffered from PTSD or Post-traumatic Stress Disorder. When a person is exposed to a horrendous event that involves the threat of death, serious injury or threat to the physical integrity of themselves or others, the intense fear, horror and helplessness involved can lead to the development of PTSD. Some of the symptoms of PTSD are flashbacks, bad dreams, feeling like the event is still happening, persistent avoidance of people, places, thoughts and feelings associated with the trauma which causes slight amnesia and increased arousal (insomnia, hyper vigilance and irritability).

In a normal memory, the memory would be integrated and reinterpreted. This process happens automatically without any input from the conscious mind and allows for the experience to be integrated with other life events.[1] In cases of PTSD, the integration process fails and the memory remains undigested and raw. In fact, the entire Central Nervous System can be reorganized based upon the traumatic experience of major harm to self or others. In cases of PTSD, the worldview can be reorganized to view the world as dangerous, self as helpless and others as a threat to the trauma victim's well being. Further PTSD causes the stress response system to remain hyper vigilant against any potential harm while the amygdala in the brain is prepared for fight or flight at any moment. The person with an unresolved trauma lives on edge, in fear and prepared for the next trauma to come.

Memories regarding traumatic events can be solidly imprinted in the mind because of the role of adrenaline. When adrenaline is released in fight or flight mode, the hormone acts to engrave the memory into our mind in a more deliberate manner than a normal experience would. In fact, the more adrenaline secreted in the moment of trauma, the more precise the memory will be.[2] During an ordinary experience, the rational and emotional brain can collaborate to have an integrated response. However, when trauma occurs and a person feels the sense of inescapable shock, areas in the brain will disconnect and the integration process will fail. The hippocampus, thalamus and other regions in the brain involved in creating meaning from an experience, storing a memory and integrating a memory shut down and fail in extreme cases of trauma.[3]

In other cases of trauma, amnesia and even dissociation can occur after an extremely traumatic experience if the trauma victim experiences inescapable shock, collapse or a freeze response. If someone lacks a verbal memory, they may repeat the trauma as an action without knowing that this is their way of remembering.[4] In the Lancet, a study was published after the British army was rescued from the beaches of Dunkirk in 1940. This study found that 10% of soldiers who were rescued suffered major memory loss after the evacuation. Delayed recall of trauma and partial or complete amnesia can be common after trauma. In fact, memory loss is one symptom of Post-traumatic Stress Disorder (PTSD) within the diagnostic criteria. In addition, there are hundreds of scientific publications that document repressed memories resurfacing years or decades after the traumatic incident.[5] In 19-38% of cases of childhood sexual abuse, the victims experienced total memory loss.[6]

Dr. Linda Meyer Williams performed a study on repressed memories and trauma starting in the 1970s. Researchers in this study followed 206 girls 10-12 years of age for 17 years starting when they were admitted to the hospital after sexual abuse occurred. Williams was able to follow up with 136 of the 206 original participants who were now adults to conduct follow up interviews. In the interviews, Williams discovered that 38% of the women did not recall the abuse with12% insisting that they were never abused. However, 68% reported other incidents of childhood sexual abuse.

Women who were younger at the time of the incident and who were molested by someone that they knew were more likely to have no memory. Further, 16% reported that they had forgotten about the abuse at some point in the past, but remembered it at a later time. Those who had a period of time where they forgot the trauma were younger at the time of the abuse and less likely to receive support from their mothers.[7]

At the time of the study, researchers found that 85% could verbally share a coherent story of the traumatic incident with a beginning, middle and an end. However, all participants shared that right after the trauma occurred, they were overwhelmed by images, sounds, sensations and emotions. As time went on, more sensory details and feelings were activated. In addition, some were able to make sense of what happened, integrate the traumatic experience and develop a story with a beginning, middle and an end. However, there were 5 participants in the study whose memories as an adult still arrived as images, physical sensations and intense emotions. These 5 participants had abusive childhoods along with the sexual abuse and could not tell a cohesive story of their past.

When a memory is inaccessible, the mind is unable to make meaning from the experience or modify the interpretation of the experience. However, when memories are retrieved, the memory can be returned to the mind with modifications and new meaning.[8] Remembering a trauma does not necessarily resolve it, but it does make it easier to move through a healing process. Finding the appropriate words and expression to what happened during and after a traumatic experience, can be transformative to a point. Many study participants could tell a coherent story, but still experienced immense pain associated with the story. And some participants were still haunted by unbearable images and physical sensations.

When trauma victims become speechless, the language area in the brain is literally shut down.[9] When I worked as a counselor in Cape Town, South

Africa I struggled to counsel severely traumatized individuals that had little or no ability to connect with their inner world, talk about their past or share their emotions. Nigel was the perfect example; he was always doing "licker, ma'am, licker." Which means really good in Afrikaans. There was never a time that he was not doing "really good."

Many years later, I reflect back on my time as a counselor in that environment and I realize that many of the students suffered from a condition called alexithymia. Brain imaging studies on trauma have found abnormal activation of the insula. The insula integrates and interprets input from internal organs, muscles, joints and balance to generate a general sense of being embodied. Further, the insula transmits signals to the amygdala, which in turn triggers fight or flight responses in a situation of stress.

After an experience of trauma, a person may not have any conscious recognition of how they are feeling. The abnormal activity of the insula will cause the person to feel on edge, unable to focus with a general sense of impending doom. Many times, the person does not connect these feelings with their original experience of trauma. Thus, the overactive insula causes the person to feel cut off from bodily sensations and can result in the development of alexithymia.

Those with alexithymia are unable to sense or communicate what is occurring within their inner world. Alexithymia can be connected with dissociation, a general sense of being shut down or out of body. Alexithymia and dissociation can lead to a major disconnect in emotional awareness and emotional intelligence. When we don't know how we feel, we can be inhibited in our ability to act upon our feelings and protect ourselves from further trauma.

In this sense, the result of an unprocessed trauma allows for a person to feel disconnected from reality, spacey and even out of body. When someone lives with unresolved trauma, the lack of integration of the memory causes a duality of reality with part of the person stuck in the trauma, reliving it over and over again and part of the person trying to survive day by day in a body that feels like it is not their own.

The area of the brain that perceives time and interprets an individual's perception of reality can be disconnected during an experience of trauma. In this case, it becomes impossible to discern between past and present realities. Taking a pendulant approach with trauma victims can help them find ways to ground themselves emotionally when the trauma becomes overwhelming to their bodily sensations.[10]

Trauma victims need to start at the foundation of building self-awareness in order to connect to their internal reality. The system in the brain devoted to self-awareness is the Medial Prefrontal Cortex or MPC. When activated appropriately, the MPC can begin to change the emotional brain. Being able to perceive bodily sensations is the foundation to emotional awareness. When we feel safe with another person and don't feel rushed, we can find the words to communicate moment-to-moment self-awareness.

Things can begin to change when we activate our internal perceptions to respond to our gut feelings, listen to our own heartbreak and follow interoceptive pathways to the inmost recesses of our being.

In 1986, Pennebaker of The University of Texas in Austin performed an interesting study on writing and trauma. He created 3 different groups of students who received the following instructions: The first group was told to write about what was currently happening in their lives. The second group was told to write the details of the most traumatic and stressful event that occurred in their lives. The third group was told to recount the details of the trauma along with three added features: how they felt, how they feel now and how the trauma impacted their lives.

Each group of participants was told to write 15-minutes per day for 4 days in a row. There were 200 students in this study. Many students wrote about the death of a family member. Another 22% of women and 10% of men wrote about sexual trauma that occurred prior to 17 years of age.[11] Those who reported sexual trauma had been hospitalized 1.7 days on average in the previous year. This was 2-fold the rate of hospitalization for the other students. Further, those who reported sexual abuse experienced higher rates of cancer, high blood pressure, ulcers, flu, headaches and earaches.

The third group who wrote in depth about the incident including their feelings and perception of the trauma had a 50% drop in doctors' visits after writing their deepest thoughts and feelings about the experience. Further, the third group experienced improved moods, a more optimistic attitude and overall better physical health at the end of the study.

A second study by Pennebaker compared the experience of 72 students. The first group spoke verbally into a tape recorder about the most traumatic experience of their lives while the control group discussed their plans for the rest of the day. Researchers monitored blood pressure, heart rate, muscle tension and hand temperature. Those who allowed themselves to feel their emotions demonstrated significant physiological changes. Those talking about traumatic experiences had a significant spike of blood pressure, heart rate and other autonomic functions during the recall of the trauma. After sharing their stories into the tape recorders, their levels dropped below where they had been at the beginning of the study. Further, the drop in blood pressure could still be measured 6 weeks after the experiment ended.[12]

Most writing studies of PTSD patients have been inconclusive. However, the studies done by Pennebaker demonstrated conclusive evidence that writing and speaking about trauma can cause physiological changes in the body. Most of the studies looking at PTSD patients had the participants sharing about trauma in a group setting after they wrote their personal stories. Perhaps, the participants in those studies did not feel the freedom needed to share their deepest trauma in the most honest, cathartic manner. Some people would feel afraid to share their deepest trauma in a group setting and would potentially change the story or pick an experience that wasn't deeply traumatic because of general mistrust or fear of the group's perception of them.

Thus, it appears that the most beneficial approach to using writing as an opportunity to heal from trauma is a private exercise in the safety of a person's own personal diary or journal that will not be viewed by other people. The best form of writing for healing after trauma is free association journaling. In free association journaling, you dump all of your thoughts and feelings without editing, judging or changing what comes to you. The object of writing to heal from trauma is to write about yourself in a way that allows you to discover what you have been trying to avoid. We will give you an opportunity to do some writing exercises on trauma at the end of this section in your companion workbook.

What does someone do when they cannot remember any trauma from their past? Or what does someone do when they find it impossible to pinpoint their emotions? The majority of my students in Cape Town would not know what to do with a writing exercise on the topic of trauma. In these cases, a body-based approach to healing in the beginning can help to calm the stress response system to allow the person to become more connected to their bodily sensations.

Further, the capacity of art, music and dance to circumvent the speechlessness-surrounding trauma is the reason that these approaches are used as trauma treatments around the world. In one study on dance and trauma, participants were placed into 3 different groups. The first group shared their traumatic experience through expressive dance movements for 10 minutes a day for 3 consecutive days. Next, they were told to write about their experience with trauma for 10 minutes a day for 3 consecutive days. In the second group, participants danced their trauma, but did not write about it. In the third group, the control group, participants performed routine exercises every day. All three groups reported feeling happier and healthier. However, the first group who danced and wrote about their past trauma had better objective physical health improvements as well as an improved grade point average.[13]

There are many effective strategies to help with the integration and processing of traumatic memories. In my practice, I use Core Belief Therapy and redesigning memories to deal with the aftermath of trauma. This book along with the workbook is another tool for my clients to navigate how to connect, process and release emotions regarding the aftermath of trauma. I hope this book and workbook guides you through past trauma and emotional pain in a way that allows you to release the negative imprint on your biology.

One therapy that has been used to integrate traumatic memories is EMDR therapy. EMDR is eye movement desensitization and reprocessing therapy. This therapy allows a person to access their memories without being overwhelmed by them. A study compared the use of Prozac to EMDR and found that for those participants who had PTSD and were depressed, EMDR was more effective at treating depression than Prozac.[14]

EMDR is related to the rapid eye movements in REM sleep cycles. The REM sleep cycles are the phases of sleep in which dreaming occurs. When we spend more time in REM sleep, the likelihood of developing depression reduces.[15] Further, PTSD is connected to disturbed sleep. Veterans with PTSD frequently wake themselves up after going into REM sleep cycles.[16]

Deep REM sleep plays a role in how memories change over time. The sleeping brain reshapes memories by increasing the imprint of emotionally relevant information while helping irrelevant material fade away.[17] Further, studies have found that the sleeping brain can make sense of memories whose relevance is unclear while we are awake, and integrate them into a larger memory system.[18] EMDR takes advantage of sleep dependent processes, which may be blocked or ineffective in those with PTSD to allow effective memory processing and trauma resolution.[19]

A study performed at The National Institute of Mental Health placed 88 subjects in 3 different groups: EMDR, Prozac and the placebo group. This PTSD study lasted for 8 weeks to compare the results of EMDR treatments to Prozac. The placebo group experienced 42% improvement, which is typical of a PTSD diagnosis. The Prozac group fared slightly better than the placebo group. The group who received 8 EMDR sessions experienced the following results: 1

in 4 were completely cured and PTSD levels dropped to negligible levels.

Further, 8 months later, 60% of those who received the 8 EMDR sessions were completely cured of PTSD. Only 10% of participants in the Prozac group experienced PTSD levels drop to negligible levels.[20] Adults with histories of childhood trauma responded very differently to EMDR than those who experienced trauma as adults.

At the end of 8 weeks, almost 50% of adult trauma victims were completely cured of PTSD, but only 9% of those who experienced childhood trauma had pronounced improvement. Eight months later, 73% of adult trauma victims were cured of PTSD whereas only 25% of those who experienced histories of child abuse resolved PTSD symptoms. Thus, EMDR is powerful for stuck traumatic memories, but doesn't resolve the effects of betrayal and abandonment that occurs with physical and sexual abuse during childhood.

Thankfully, redesigning memories in a targeted way with Core Belief Therapy addresses the deeper issues of childhood abuse and trauma. There is always hope and there is always a way to resolve unresolved trauma. A specific approach to healing from trauma like EMDR may work well for one trauma victim, while not working well for another trauma victim.

There are many potential strategies to overcoming childhood trauma and adult trauma beyond Core Belief Therapy, EMDR, dance, massage, music and other therapies that we have already explored. First and foremost, a person who has experienced trauma must be willing to open up to a messy, painful process of healing. Unfortunately, to heal from trauma, we must feel the uncomfortable sensations and emotional pain involved with the trauma. Secondly, loving connection found in relationships and community can help a person process past trauma. "The roots of resilience are to be found in the sense of being understood by and existing in the mind and heart of a loving, attuned, and self-possessed other (Diana Fosha)."

Thirdly, attachment bonds to a primary caregiver can be the greatest protection against the long-term negative effects of trauma.[21] Studies conducted during WWII found that children who lived in London during German bombing raids, but stayed with parents in the bomb shelters recovered from the trauma of war better than children who were sent away to the countryside to stay with families for protection. The children who stayed with their parents in bombing shelters were exposed to graphic images of destroyed buildings and dead people. Yet, they were able to recover from trauma better because they remained with their primary caregiver to whom they were securely attached.

Safe and protective early relationships are crucial to protect children from long-term problems associated with childhood trauma. Equally, trauma that occurs in the context of relationships with primary caregivers are much more difficult to resolve than trauma from traffic accidents or natural disasters. If the people you rely on for care and protection terrify, abandon, abuse and reject you, you learn to shut down and ignore what you feel.[22] In cases of child abuse, molestation, incest, rape and domestic violence, children find alternative ways to deal with fear, anger and frustration. In order to survive these horrific experiences, children can learn to dissociate or experiment with drugs and alcohol to self-medicate rather than face the chronic emotional pain and despair. Trauma in childhood with primary caregivers ultimately results in a breakdown of attuned physical synchrony and relationships begin to be marked by alienation, disconnect, fear and mistrust.

In fact, researchers at McGill discovered that abused children in both privileged and poor economic situations had the same modifications in 73 genes as a result of the abuse. Researchers concluded the following: "Major changes to our bodies can be made not just by chemicals and toxins, but also in the way that the social world talks to the hard-wired world."[23] In the same respect, genetic vulnerability and flaws can be protected with appropriate support and parenting skills.

There are 2 variants of the serotonin gene, the short or long serotonin transporter allele. In humans, the short allele has been associated with impulsivity, aggression, sensation seeking, suicide attempts and severe depression. Monkeys share these same genetic varieties as humans. A study on monkeys explored the serotonin gene and how genes are affected by parental attachments. Researchers discovered that monkeys who genetically received the short serotonin allele who were raised by an adequate mother behaved normally with no deficit in serotonin metabolism. However, those monkeys who had the short serotonin allele who were raised inadequately by peer monkeys became aggressive risk takers.[24] Alec Roy, a New Zealand researcher, found that humans with the short serotonin allele had increased rates of depression, but only if they had a history of childhood abuse or neglect.

Ying Mee arrived in the United States at 5 years of age from China with no ability to communicate. She had been raised in an orphanage and became mute before being adopted. Ying Mee could not resonate with voices and the faces of people around her. She was exposed to a sensory integration clinic where she physically engaged her environment in play. She jumped in a tub of plastic balls, swayed on swings, crawled under weighted blankets and performed many other playful and creative explorations. After 6 weeks of immersion in the Sensory Integration Clinic in Watertown, Massachusetts, Ying Mee began to talk and was no longer mute.[25]

Now it is your opportunity to explore past trauma in the companion workbook. Use this opportunity to discover what is necessary to heal and resolve past, unresolved trauma that may be hindering your body and biochemistry from expressing health.

Section 3: Unraveling the Imprint of Trauma

Chapter 5: Healing the Abandoned Heart

My heart sank as I stepped into the room and saw a dozen or so babies lying on their backs with their eyes wide open and their arms flailing. They both broke and captured my heart at the same time. I quickly scanned the room and saw workers either calloused or oblivious to the vulnerable cries of the babies. I saw one small baby girl out of the corner of my eye that captured my attention. She couldn't have been more than 2 months old and she showed no signs of distress, as her eyes and face were free of emotion. A sign of neglect, weeks of crying led to no relief, so this baby girl simply stopped giving necessary cues in order to save energy and survive. I quickly picked her up and held her close to my chest. She was to be my baby for the duration of my time at the orphanage.

Every day, I went to the orphanage to find my baby, Anam. Every couple of days, I would see small improvement, until I started to see expressions of emotion on her face and her being able to recognize me. Bonding with one adult consistently while having workers respond to her needs for food, attention and diaper changes allowed Anam to slowly transition out of survival mode. A few months later, we started to see her sparkly, funny personality emerge. She began to win the hearts of every volunteer who came to work at the orphanage with her uncanny ability to ignite laughter and joy to those around her.

After the summer wrapped up, I began to volunteer as a counselor at the high school for at-risk youth that was literally around the corner and started to spend less time at the orphanage. One day, I went to see Anam. Clearly angry with me, Anam began to grimace her face at me and hit me over and over again. I understood perfectly what she was saying, "You left me, why would you leave me, too?" Again, my heart broke into a thousand pieces for this little girl. I desired to continue the bond that we had, but I knew that open adoption was not possible. At the time, South African laws kept adoption within the country and preferably within the family or culture of origin.

The plight of an orphaned child was outside of my realm of understanding prior to my work at the non-profit in Cape Town. Being in the midst of the tragic needs of HIV/AIDS orphaned babies made me feel completely helpless and desperate to help at the same time. How could one person help the plight of millions of orphaned children around the world? All I could do is help one baby at a time. It felt like I didn't have enough to meet the overwhelming needs around me.

After 7 months of working at the orphanage and school for at-risk youth, my visa was expiring and I had a plane ticket home. In my heart of hearts, I knew that I would be back. South Africa became my second home. I also had found another piece of my identity puzzle; I wanted to fund orphanage work and make a larger impact in the future. Anam had made a deep imprint on my soul. I would never forget her vulnerability and need the first day that I saw her lying on the ground, helpless and neglected. I would also never forget how she came alive with the proper care and attention at the orphanage.

The hardest thing to face before leaving South Africa was when I had to say good-bye to my baby, Anam. At that point in her journey, she had begun to thrive; her personality and physical health were both in an excellent state and I had high hopes for her future. She had a winsome personality and shared love and joy to everyone around her. I knew the orphanage was trying to find a placement for Anam within her community of origin and I could only hope for the right solution for her long-term. The orphanage was a short-term placement that sought to reconcile the child with a family from their community of origin when their parents were unable to care for their needs long-term. Many times, the parents were diagnosed with HIV/AIDS and did not have the resources or physical health necessary to care for the needs of a small infant.

It would be years later that I would again visit the orphanage and seek to find Anam. The social worker at the orphanage knew where Anam had been placed and desired to bring me to her. We drove deep into the townships within Cape Town along winding, dirt roads until we arrived at a small shack that housed Anam. The social worker went inside to retrieve Anam and I waited anxiously, wondering if she would remember me. As she came out of the house with the social worker, I felt a stabbing pain in my chest and my breathing became labored. I was on the edge of a full-on panic attack.

Anam stared at me with the same void, numb look that I saw in her eyes when she first arrived at the orphanage. Now 4 years old, the deep pain of neglect etched on her face, hardened her and made her appear years older than she was. She expressed no joy or playfulness, just the harsh look of a child who was not seen when she felt scared, not held when she was crying and not cared for when she needed basic things like food and attention. Anam was a shell of her joyful, spontaneous self and she showed no signs of remembering me. In the 30-minutes that I spent with her, I couldn't get a smile or any type of expression out of Anam; rather, she continued to look at me with this blank, dull look that left me full of pain and regret. Even today, I can still see the frown that was cemented on her face and the empty look in her eyes.

I went home from this trip to South Africa completely devastated. I cried on and off for days and struggled to communicate the depth of pain and trauma that I felt in being reunited with Anam. I think about Anam often. My resolve to help orphaned, abandoned and neglected children has only strengthened in the passing of time as I reflect on my baby Anam and how the system failed her.

While I may never understand the childhood trauma that someone like Anam has endured, I have an immense amount of compassion for her tragic story. What allows some people to overcome the most intense forms of trauma while others flounder and may never recover from a childhood full of pain? There may be several key factors that I have outlined in this book for you: the lack of honesty, introspection, emotional intelligence, the lack of communal support, the lack of understanding and the lack of focus on redemptive purpose. We will speak more about redemptive purpose in Section 4, for now let's look at a few more innovative approaches to healing from trauma.

In 1924, a German psychiatrist, Hansberger, developed a new technology called electroencephalography or EEG.[1] Hansberger discovered that different brain wave patterns would reflect different mental activities. For example, when someone is solving a math problem, the frequency band beta is released at high levels. EEG patterns have also been found to correlate with different mental problems. In fact, the EEG has been used to diagnose seizure activity in epilepsy.

In 2013, slow-wave prefrontal activity became a biomarker for ADHD. For those with ADHD, brain waves were slow in the prefrontal cortex which would lead to poor executive functioning, a lack of control over the emotional brain and an increase in hyper-vigilance surrounding potential stressors in the environment.[2]

In a study on PTSD, Alexander McFarlene discovered key differences between how people with trauma processed information versus how people without trauma processed information.[3] In the control group, which consisted of Australians who did not experience trauma, key parts of the brain worked together to produce a coherent pattern of filtering focus while analyzing information. However, the brain waves of those with a traumatic past were loosely coordinated and failed to develop a coherent pattern of activity. The mind of the participants with trauma could not generate brain wave patterns that would allow for them to pay attention to a task at hand by filtering out irrelevant information. Further, core information-processing configuration of the brain was poorly defined. This explains why traumatized individuals have trouble learning from experience and struggle to fully engage in day-to-day life. Their brains are not organized to pay careful attention to what is happening in the present moment.

Neurofeedback is a brain treatment that can help to address this type of disorganization of the brain. Neurofeedback treatments help the brain to adjust its frequencies in order to create new patterns that enhance its natural complexity and its bias towards self-regulation.[4] Neurofeedback intervenes in the circuitry that promotes states of fear, shame and rage and helps to change habitual brain patterns created by trauma. When fear patterns in the brain relax, the brain becomes less susceptible to automatic stress reactions and can better focus on ordinary events.

Neurofeedback can stabilize the brain and help to increase resiliency.

One thing that I noticed working as a counselor at the school for at-risk youth was the fact that the majority of the students struggled to learn. They would blankly stare at their teachers and write on their desks or pants instead of taking notes. Intuitively, I felt that the students were unable to learn because of the unresolved trauma, neglect, abuse and violence in their pasts. Sometimes, I felt that the focus of the school should be on resolving trauma first, which would allow the students to learn and excel in studies like normal students.

Quite literally, trauma changes your brain waves. A person who suffered trauma in the past has excessive activity in their right temporal lobe, the fear center of the brain. Also, trauma victims have excessive slow-wave activity in their frontal lobes, which leads to symptoms reminiscent of ADHD. The emotional brains dominate their mental life and people with a history of trauma struggle to absorb new information in a normal manner. Chronic abuse and neglect in childhood interfere with the proper wiring of sensory integration systems and can result in faulty connections between auditory and word-processing systems, poor hand-eye coordination, poor learning skills and difficulty processing day-to-day information. Thus, trauma and neglect can be disguised as learning disabilities or behavioral problems in school. When trauma is appropriately addressed, the learning disability, behavioral problem or ADHD symptoms may disappear.

Neurofeedback has been found to decrease PTSD scores, improve mental clarity and increase a person's capacity to regulate how upset he or she becomes in response to minor problems. In addition, 36 studies have shown that neurofeedback is as effective as drugs in treating ADHD without any side effects. The neurofeedback treatments have helped to enhance focus, attention and concentration.[5]

Alpha/theta training with neurofeedback has helped traumatic events to be re-interpreted in the mind. In the alpha/theta training, theta waves help the mind to focus on the internal world while alpha waves act as a bridge from the external world to the internal world. Theta activity helps to loosen conditioned connections between stimuli that evoke an emotional trigger while the mind enters into a trance-like state. In this state, the mind can make new associations to traumatic memories. For example, the sound of gun shots can lose their trigger to trauma and instead of being associated to violence and death, gun shots can be associated with fireworks on the 4th of July.[6]

Eugene Penistron and Paul Kulkosky used neurofeedback to treat 29 Vietnam veterans with a 12-15-year history of combat related PTSD. Half of the men were treated with EEF alpha/theta training whereas half were treated with psychotropic drugs and therapy. The group treated with neurofeedback was instructed to recline back in their recliners with their eyes closed while being coached to allow neurofeedback sounds to guide them into deep relaxation. In this state, their brains would increase alpha and theta wave activity.

The group treated with neurofeedback experienced a significant decrease in PTSD symptoms, physical complaints, depression, anxiety as well as paranoia.[7] At the 30-month follow-up after the study completed, only 3 of the 15 participants reported disturbing flashbacks and nightmares, only 1 needed to go to the hospital for further treatments and 14 out of 15 participants used significantly less medications. In the control group, all 14 veterans experienced an increase in symptoms of PTSD, each participant required 2 hospitalizations in the 30-month period after the study and 10 of the 14 veterans needed an increase in their medications.[8]

Statistically speaking, one-third to one-half of traumatized people will develop substance abuse problems.[9] Drugs and alcohol provide temporary relief from trauma symptoms but as soon as drugs and alcohol are stopped, there is an increase in hyper-arousal, nightmares, flashbacks and irritability.

Penistron and Kulkosky performed a study exploring the impact of neurofeedback treatments on alcoholism. Half of the study group received alpha/theta neurofeedback training and the control group received standard treatments. After 3 years, 8 of the 15 participants in the neurofeedback group stopped drinking completely, most were less depressed, more warm-hearted, more intelligent, more emotionally stable, more socially bold, more relaxed and more satisfied with their lives. However, the group who received the standard of care did not have good results. In fact, all participants in the control group were re-admitted to the hospital within 18 months of the study.[10]

Neurofeedback is a powerful treatment tool that can be used to support those recovering from trauma when other forms of treatment have failed. Since trauma causes areas of the brain to shut down, activating different parts of the brain by creating opportunities to express emotions, energy and artistic creativity can help in shifting the brain towards healing. Journaling, meditation, dance, song, musical expression, chorus, Pilates, spoken word and theater can help a person with a history of trauma to connect and release deep emotions.

In South Africa, Desmond Tutu conducted public hearings where witness's recounted unspeakable atrocities inflicted upon them. When the witness would be overcome with emotion, Tutu would lead the entire audience in prayer, song and dance until the witness could contain their sobbing. This was a healing moment for a nation divided by years of legalized segregation, racial abuse, discriminatory laws and practices by the Apartheid regime.

A 2,500-year-old play called *The Theater of War 2,500* gives voice to the plight of combat veterans and fosters dialogue and understanding between veterans and loved ones.[11] After the play, a town hall style discussion allows veterans to share what they experienced in war, to identify with parts of the play and to connect with friends and family members in a unique way to foster compassion and understanding to the trauma they endured through war.

There are theater treatment programs in Boston, Massachusetts and New York City called Urban Improv, Trauma Drama, The Possibility Project and Shakespeare in the Courts. These treatment theater programs allow at-risk youth to confront painful realities in their lives, express deep emotions and undergo symbolic transformation through communal action.[12] Acting provides an opportunity to connect and convey intense emotions to an audience. This is very critical to traumatized individuals who are many times fearful of deep emotions that hijack their minds when past trauma is triggered.

Theater gives an opportunity for people dealing with trauma to become aware of their emotions, to give voice to those emotions, to come out of isolation into community and to experience rhythmic syncing with other individuals. Further, conflict is central to theater and people with trauma struggle to face relational and internal conflicts directly. In theater, traumatized individuals practice facing inner conflicts, interpersonal conflicts, family conflicts and social conflicts while learning potential strategies that they can apply to their own personal conflicts. And lastly, theater allows for an opportunity to develop competence in a skill set. Competence in anything is the best defense against the helplessness of trauma.

After my sweet baby, Noble Thomas died during labor and delivery, I felt like my arm had been amputated and I never knew if I would feel normal again. The ripple effect of trauma stole my breath and my mind and caused me to be hyper-vigilant against any potential threats to my well being and the well being of loved ones.

Today, when I meet people devastated with the loss of a child, I want to share my story and give hope of the possibility of recovery from trauma. I remember moments of pouring out my heart, my tears and the depths of my grief, just to face it again hours later as I recounted the tragedy to my community. One day in January of 2017, six months after Noble died, I noticed that I couldn't even think about the possibility of getting pregnant and having another child. In fact, I pushed it away from my mind, deciding that I would contemplate getting pregnant again in about 5 years. During my grieving process, I more deeply invested my time and energies into my passion of working with cancer patients. I felt competent and satisfied by the challenge and reward of my work and it eased the dull pain and helplessness of losing my son.

I was terrified to get pregnant again and face labor and delivery. I didn't know if I could survive the loss of another child or the trauma evoked by the natural process of labor and delivery. This is when a miracle happened. I went to sleep one night and woke up after the most vivid, transformative dream I have ever had. In the dream, I was pregnant and went into labor very quickly. While I was in labor, I thought to myself, "This is so different than the first time." I quickly and easily gave birth to a baby girl. I was full of joy as I looked down at my baby girl smiling at me. I woke up with that image burned into my mind. An hour or so later, I received a call from my midwife, Jessica, who wanted to know how I was doing. I hadn't heard from her in about 5 months.

That afternoon, I received a call from a woman who was considering taking my CPU course. After speaking for 20-minutes or so, without prompting or previous knowledge, she started to share her story of losing 3 children and then giving birth to 3 beautiful babies. That evening, I was overwhelmed with emotion and peace. I felt a shift in my heart. Suddenly, I had a strong desire to get pregnant; whereas, only 24-hours previously, I didn't want to think about the possibility of becoming pregnant for 5 years. I had just witnessed a miraculous transformation in my experience of trauma and the transformation was triggered by a vivid dream.

The loss of my child has become a distant memory that feels like another lifetime. This is the type of transformation that I believe we can all experience. In order to experience transformational restoration after trauma, we need to courageously face the depths of emotional pain, loss, despair and fear while opening our minds and hearts to internal, communal and spiritual connection that allows for a new expression of wholeness. The dream that I had resulted from a new sense of spiritual connection that developed after my son died. The next section of this book will give you more insight into spiritual connection and allow an opportunity for you to experience spiritual growth and transformation. I encourage the reader to be open to new possibilities, to challenging old mindsets and paradigms that exclude a spiritual reality in order to experience the spiritual realm in a transformative manner.

Now, open your companion workbook and complete the questions and exercises regarding trauma. Just like I experienced resolve in the most traumatic experience in my life, losing Noble, I believe that you are on your way to trauma being completely resolved in your heart and mind.

Section 4: Wakefulness

Chapter 1: Wake up to Spiritual Reality

Self-reflection doesn't always result in life-changing epiphanies, which may be why some people disengage from the tedious process altogether. Some days I journal, meditate and attempt to connect with myself and nothing appears to happen. In fact, I remember days that I would almost fall asleep or feel bored by the daily ritual that I created in my life. However, the days that the revelation finally comes makes the days of habitual pursuit worth it.

One of those days I can still picture and feel the palpable emotions involved. This epiphany changed the course of my pursuit. I was young, 16 or 17 years old and I was sitting on a couch in my basement. I remember eating ice cream while reflecting on my life. I evaluated each area of my life: relationships, finances, school, achievements and sports. I had good friendships in my life and a circle of friends with whom I could both laugh and have serious conversations. I played 3 sports in high school and performed decently enough to letter in all of the sports that I pursued including hockey, volleyball and track. I thoroughly enjoyed being part of a team, feeling a sense of belonging that gave me a purpose greater than myself. I excelled tremendously in school and had a 4.0 grade point average with an A in every class. Perfect record. Also, I had enrolled in many AP classes to prepare for college and to test out of various college courses.

Continuing to drift deeper into my reflection, I thought about my resume. I had a very good resume that would open the door to a variety of excellent and well-renewed universities, perhaps even Ivy League schools. My future was very promising as a result. My dad owned a business and money was never an issue for our family. Anything that I ever needed or wanted would be easily provided for and paying for college was not a concern. My future was also financially secured. I had been raised in a good family with loving, devoted parents and two older brothers who were my friends.

And yet, I floundered at the end of the assessment of my life because the deep sense that I felt after examining every area in my life was this: an endless vacuum of nothingness. I felt empty and devoid of purpose. My life was meaningless. What was I missing? And what would bring me meaning and fulfillment? Most people would have looked at my life on the outside and thought that I felt a great sense of significance and even happiness, but all I could find was a desperate sense of emptiness.

This was the beginning of a new pursuit for me. I needed to find the answer to that deep sense of emptiness in my soul. I felt pulled towards fulfilling an existential void of purpose that evaded me in all of my selfish ambition and pursuits. It would take me several years to realize the depth of what I was missing, but I look back at that moment in my life as the beginning of something new growing in my heart. I was turning towards spiritual meaning and the search for a deep spiritual connection.

Viktor Frankl was a Viennese personality therapist that often debated Freud. Frankl contended that man's primary need was to experience a deep sense of meaning and purpose in their life. Freud believed that the primary need of man was to seek pleasure. Frankl postulated that when meaning could not be found that man would seek pleasure instead. He further believed and advocated for life to be structured in a way that people could experience meaning. He had three main recommendations in his Logotherapy or therapy of meaning:[1]

1. Have a project to work on every day, a reason to get out of bed in the morning and something that serves a need for others. If your job or career doesn't immediately give meaning, develop something within your job or outside of your job to feed the need to have significance in your life.
2. Have a redemptive perspective on life's challenges. When something traumatic happens in your life, find ways to pursue meaning or redemption in the midst of suffering.

3. Share your life with a person or a community of people who love you unconditionally.

Frankl was in charge of the mental health division of a Viennese hospital system. At one point, his division carried more than 30,000 suicidal patients. He approached their care using Logotherapy as outlined above. Community groups were created and counselors were taught to identify projects that the patients could contribute to that would serve others and give the patient meaning in their life. Frankl had patients write down the most difficult experiences in their lives, expressing their pain at the same time that they were instructed to reflect and write down any positives that came out of their painful experience. Following the principles of Logotherapy, Frankl had not one patient commit suicide.[2] This is astounding and demonstrates the intrinsic need for everyone to make a significant contribution along with finding redemptive perspective in the face of tragedy.

At John Hopkins University, a study was performed that followed 1,337 medical students to examine personality traits and internal emotional processing habits and how they contributed to the development of disease. Dr. Caroline Thomas at John Hopkins University Medical School took personality profiles of these medical students starting in 1946. Every year after 1946, she continued to survey their mental and physical health for decades after graduation. Her goal was to find psychological precursors to heart disease, high blood pressure, mental illness and suicide.

She included cancer simply for comparison sake, not thinking there was any psychological component to cancer. However, she discovered something shocking about cancer and suicide. The traits of those who developed cancer were seemingly identical to those who later committed suicide.[3] All of the cancer patients throughout their lives restricted their emotions and had aggressive emotions related to their own needs being suppressed. Those who later committed suicide also operated with the internal emotional processing habit of restricting their emotions. Further, similar to those who developed cancer, they carried aggressive emotions to their own needs being suppressed as well.

The 30,000 suicidal patients under the care of Frankl did not commit suicide. They were actively engaged in a process of developing their purpose and finding a way to make a meaningful contribution to others. Further, they were developing their purpose in a community setting while examining personal trauma in the light of redemptive outcomes. I have always found it ominous and sad that the recommendation when someone is having suicidal tendencies is for the therapist to ask their patient to agree to call and share that they are going to act out their plan to commit suicide. Those who reach out and tell someone about their plan to commit suicide are much less likely to follow through. The shame, emotional pain and regret that are involved in a person contemplating suicide are uncovered in the act of sharing that plan with someone else. And the communal support lifts the shame and isolation that many times invokes someone to commit suicide.

I haven't had a lot of experience with friends and family members committing suicide. However, I have been to the funerals of two people in my community who did commit suicide. Both situations were absolutely heart wrenching. My high school friend, Dave, and I had just reconnected at an addiction recovery group. I was volunteering as a counselor and he had been through the program and was transitioning to the role of a volunteer. At the time we reconnected, Dave was pursuing a deeper spiritual connection and was trying to find more meaning in his life.

We went out to dinner together to catch up. One part of the interaction always stuck out to me. At the end, we were deciding whether or not to split a dessert. Dave agonized over the decision like he was deciding whether or not to move out of the country. He agonized over what he would feel like afterwards, what the sugar would do to his body and how damaging it would be to the cells in his body. In the end, he decided to split the chocolate cake with me. After we enjoyed the cake, Dave spent several more minutes talking about how much he regretted his decision to order the dessert. I made a mental note to never share a dessert with him again and moved on with my life, not thinking much about it afterwards.

Weeks later, another friend from high school, Britt, called me and uttered the shocking phrase, "Dave committed suicide this weekend." In shock, I racked my brain for a time that Dave shared that he was struggling with depression or suicidal tendencies. I couldn't think of anything. In fact, I didn't remember him talking about his emotions at all. All I could think about was that damn chocolate cake and why it was such a dilemma for Dave to eat that dessert with me. And then it hit me. That was the problem. Dave didn't tell anyone he was struggling with depression or sadness. He suffered in the prison of his own making and didn't allow anyone to help him. He wasn't able to share his deep emotions in a way to normalize his dark days. As a result, he didn't realize that everyone struggled emotionally and mentally from time to time. He was attempting to be perfect and he was failing every day without realizing that everyone else was too. The only difference was that everyone else had someone in their lives to share their feelings of pain, failure and regret.

The commonality between Dave* and the other person in my community who committed suicide, Josh* (*I changed both of their names to protect their families) was this: perfectionistic tendencies with nobody to share their imperfections and vulnerabilities to. Josh told no one of his plan to commit suicide. When he was found, it was clear that he had been planning it for a while. Josh also had perfectionist tendencies. I remember going out to eat with his family and watching him cut his steak into tiny, bite-sized portions, chewing each piece for 5 minutes at a time. He would always be the last one done eating. He was very calculating. But he was also hurting.

279

Unfortunately, he didn't want to be a "softy" and open up about his pain and where he felt that he had failed in life to anyone that would judge him and make him feel weak.

The night before the funeral of Dave, Britt had a dream that Dave was smiling and waving at us from eternity. She decided to tell his mother to try to bring her some comfort that Dave was okay on the other side of eternity even if he wasn't okay in this life. I couldn't imagine the agony of a mother, father, spouse or sibling who lost their loved one to suicide. No one knew that Dave was contemplating suicide or that he struggled with depression. He could never open up the depths of his emotional struggle and the weight of his deep sense of being flawed.

The ironic thing about sharing your flaws to another human being is that once you open up your weaknesses, flaws and mistakes to the right person, at the right time, they seem to be swallowed up by the loving acceptance of a compassionate listener. I remember sharing my deep sense of feeling flawed to a friend after an exercise that exposed it all to me.

My best friend Joe and I were pursuing an internship in L.A. at the time of the incident. We went to a motivational speaking event where the speaker was sharing about how to pursue a life of freedom and spiritual connection. Joe volunteered for a live exercise to demonstrate some of the strategies. I remember the motivational speaker saying many things to Joe that had personal meaning, but at one point he simply spoke out, "I break this unhealthy soul tie." As soon as he said this, I felt something break off of me. I knew that I was the other side of this unhealthy soul tie. All of a sudden, I felt empty, alone and exposed.

I spoke with my friend, Julie, afterwards and burst out crying, "I'm so messed up." She hugged me and said, "I know, I am too." It was exactly the response that I needed to feel unconditionally loved and accepted. Something shifted in me at that moment. Further, this was the beginning of a new level of wholeness for me. I didn't know the depths of how I was using my relationship with Joe to fill a void in my soul until his soul was quite literally broken off of mine.

The other strange thing about this moment appeared the next day; I noticed imperfections about Joe that I had never seen before despite knowing him intimately for four years. I saw imperfections in his face, scars and even acne that I didn't see previously. It was a perplexing moment of realization that I had been relying upon Joe for emotional and spiritual completion because I had been so incomplete and desperate for connection. I had been trying to take the easy road when the hard road demanded surrender, discipline, patience, raw honesty and a little bit of chaos while all of my issues worked out of my system.

I had a lack of spiritual awareness and spiritual connection. I had been raised in a good family with values of hard work, commitment, excellence and striving to do our best. In college, I met friends who had a deep spiritual understanding and connection and I started to desire to find that path of peace for myself.

I began a process of honest introspection in college mainly because of the incessant panic attacks that I was experiencing. I started to ask a lot of hard questions about life, death, spirituality and how to find a path of purpose. I decided to rush for a sorority at the beginning of my second semester as all of my friends were rushing and it was the main social scene at Vanderbilt. Like speed dating on steroids, rushing was a bizarre process for a Northern feminist. An introvert by nature, I was very uncomfortable with spending five minutes talking to someone and then moving onto the next person. I was the type of person who would find one person at a party and talk about deep things the whole time and then leave feeling satisfied.

At the end of "Rush Week," we were told to write down our top three sorority picks and turn it in before the day of the results. The sororities would also submit their desired picks. I was nervous the day of the results, but felt that one of my top three picks would also choose me. I went to the place where we would receive our results with my friend, MeBird. As I shared my name to the person who had my results, her face became red and I knew that something was wrong. She whispered to me, "You fell out." I didn't know what that meant, but I knew that it wasn't a good result. MeBird walked back to the dorm room with me, explaining what "falling out" meant. Softly, Mebird explained, "The sororities that you picked in your top 3, did not pick you. Falling out means that you don't have a placement for a sorority."

Tears streaming down my face, I was absolutely gutted. It felt like the entire school rejected me at that moment. I was equally devastated to find out that my friends were placed into the sororities that they desired. That weekend, MeBird slept on the floor of my dorm room and all of my friends bought me pints of Ben & Jerry's ice cream. My dad sent me a beautiful bouquet of roses with a note, "To the most beautiful girl at Vanderbilt." I felt loved and supported in that moment, but the inner turmoil raged and pushed me to the edge.

MeBird said to me with her Southern charm, "Don't you want to go to church with me on Sunday?" I told her that I would go with her. I wasn't much of a churchgoer, but I trusted my friend and I was open to learn more. That Sunday morning, MeBird picked me up in her SUV and had a dozen Krispy Kreme donuts to share. I felt slightly uncomfortable, as the church was very active with people dancing and waving flags.

I had never been around that type of religious environment. I sat in the pew and hoped that nobody noticed that I was new. As the music was playing and people were singing, I began to cry and felt the pain of the rejection run through my entire body. **All of a sudden, I felt my heart break into thousands of pieces and then I felt a hand go inside of my chest and put my heart back together. I felt complete peace for the first time in my life.** In that moment, I knew that God was real and I knew that God cared deeply about my pain. This was the start of a new understanding of the world. No longer did I feel alone in my pain, I felt like I had a friend that deeply cared about my experience on planet earth. Spirituality opened up to me like a budding flower and my life shifted towards the spiritual depth that I had desired for a long time, but it seemed to evade me.

This was the first time in my life that I felt that I could personally connect with God. I believed in some sort of God-figure, but I couldn't pinpoint my exact beliefs. Spiritual connection did not seem readily available to me, until that moment. To look at my experience in a different light, Dr. Gail Ironson at The University of Miami performed a 4-year study on HIV/AIDS and the impact of a person's belief system on their immune system response.

Dr. Ironson found that the biggest difference in the strength of the immune system response was found in those who held the belief that God was benevolent, loving and wanted a personal relationship with them. Those with HIV/AIDS who believed in a personal, benevolent God expressed stronger immune system responses with a lower viral load count found in their bloodstreams. In fact, those who did not believe that God loved them lost helper T-cells 3 times faster than those who did, their viral load increased 3-times faster and their stress levels were elevated.[4]

This study is one of many that demonstrate that our beliefs impact our biology in a profound manner. The study of epigenetics is one of the most active areas of research currently. Epigenetics means upon the gene and epigenetics research explores what aspects of a person's psychology, nutrition and lifestyle trigger genetic expression within the body. Our thoughts, emotions, beliefs and nutrition all have an ability to get under the skin of our DNA to cause either positive changes to genetic expression or negative changes to genetic expression.[5]

In fact, a study done at The Institute of HeartMath found that thinking and feeling anger, fear and frustration caused DNA to change shape. The researchers found that when participants focused on anger, fear and frustrations, DNA tightened up and became shorter whereas when the participants focused on feelings of love, joy and gratitude, DNA became looser and longer.[6]

Prior to my experience at MeBird's church, I did not believe in a God who wanted an intimate relationship with me. I would have been in the same category of people whose immune systems were weaker and stress levels were higher based upon their beliefs. No wonder why I was having panic attacks every day! My beliefs about the spiritual world being distant and impersonal made me feel alone, abandoned and on my own. Achieving something great in the world was all up to my effort and execution. The burden of my destiny and impact on the world was upon my shoulders. And it was heavy.

The depth of my belief, "I am alone and abandoned," did not surface for me until I found myself in Israel. During my trip to Israel, I experienced some of the most profound spiritual moments of my life. While meditating and journaling, I became aware of a memory in my conscious mind that I had never accessed previously. In the memory, I was in 2nd grade and I was sitting in my room playing the game "Hidden Pictures" in my favorite magazine *Highlights for Children.* It was my favorite puzzle to play and I looked forward to receiving my magazine every month to find all of the hidden pictures. On that particular day, I decided to time myself. I wanted to become the fastest person in the world at finding the hidden pictures in *Highlights for Children.*

As I examined the memory, I saw that the door was closed tightly and that there were questions on the door that kept it shut. The questions popping up on the door were questions like, "Why was I alone? Where were you? Why did I have to be alone so much?" I saw my little self in the room feeling alone with the weight of the world upon her shoulders. I understood her and I felt my heart break for her.

At that moment in time, alone in my room, my life changed because I perceived that I was abandoned. My beliefs about an impersonal, unemotional spiritual realm were solidified. It was at that time that I decided that I needed to strive and excel to become admired and seen. At school, I started to excel in math and asked for more math worksheets from my teacher to get ahead of the other students. I pushed myself to learn at a fast pace and to excel above my peers. I had to get a perfect score otherwise I was dejected and sad about my performance. But what I realized on a deeper level was that it wasn't just anyone's attention that I desired, I wanted my dad's attention.

Again, I grew up in an amazing, supportive home with loving parents. My dad loved me and felt that his role was to financially provide a secure future for his children. Sundays were my favorite day because it was the day that my dad always planned a fun outing for his children. He would take us to the A & W Root Beer stand, to Dairy Queen and all kinds of places that children love. I know with all of my heart that my parents raised us the best that they knew how and that my childhood was blessed as a result. However, I also know that no matter how great your upbringing is, there are always defining moments in childhood that can result in a negative perception about yourself, the world and spirituality.

Around the time of the "Hidden Pictures" memory, my dad bought the family business from my grandpa. He came home more tired after work and his energy was more focused around making the salvage lot a success. I felt his energy shift from home to work. I "knew" that I had to do something amazing to get his attention. Thus, I began to strive in my "Hidden Pictures" game and my worksheets at school.

The other thing that I realized about the memory was that the questions that kept the door shut were both for my dad and for God. I felt abandoned by my dad emotionally, but at the same time, I felt abandoned by God. It seems that when children are young, the spiritual realm or God is reflected to them best through the way their caregivers show love, attention and affirmation. Parents and caregivers have a God-like quality when children are growing up. Thus, the parent's ability to care for their children can reflect a loving, intimate God or it can reflect a detached, distant God. As the door shut to my room, it not only shut out the emotional intimacy that I desired with my dad, but it also shut out the possibility of an intimate, personal God.

In Israel, all of the patterns of my life began to make sense. I understood why I strived in school and had to receive a perfect score in every class. But I also came to realize why I had a codependent tendency and clung to Joe's friendship so desperately. Joe was the perfect friend to fill the void of abandonment because he was loyal, predictable and emotionally present for me. I stuck Joe into the void of my soul, the abandonment that caused me to feel so insecure and desperate for attention from men and it helped for a while. Until, it didn't. In Israel, I saw the memory and I felt the questions melt off of the door as I received intimate love from God that healed the deep void of abandonment in my soul.

Now it is time to explore your own spirituality in the companion workbook. Take time to think deeply and answer the questions surrounding meaning, purpose and spirituality. If you have never developed a strong spiritual connection, now is your chance!

Section 4: Wakefulness

Chapter 2: We all Have an Incurable Disease

My heart fluttering and my breath labored, I struggled to get ready to go and meet my parents. I wondered if I made the right decision and I felt nervous to see the results of my decision. As I felt numb and unable to process my emotions, we drove to the funeral parlor to meet my parents. The last place that I wanted to be on that particular Sunday, we pulled into the parking lot to plan a funeral for my first son, Noble.

Struggling to get out of the car, I heard myself sigh again. All kinds of spontaneous sounds of grief escaped my body at that time. Just 4 days post-partum, I waddled into the church chapel to see my son again. It had been 3 days since we said goodbye to Noble in the hospital. After Noble died, nurses came in immediately to ask us if we wanted to donate his organs. If we did, they would have to take Noble from us immediately. If we declined, Noble could stay with us for 24-hours. In shock and unable to say goodbye right away, we declined to donate his organs. We asked for the full 24-hour period allowed so that we could grieve properly. Hardly enough time to say hello and goodbye to our first son, we cried on and off, took pictures with him, had his footprints made in cement and had family and friends meet Noble and grieve with us in the hospital. When the nurse came just 24-hours later, we were overcome with grief again.

Sobbing and shaking, I said my last words of love to my first son before he was whisked away. Before we left the hospital the next day, we were asked if we wanted to do an autopsy to find out why Noble died. I had a sense that they wouldn't find anything in an autopsy and I wanted to say no. But my parents thought that we should do an autopsy in case there was something that happened that we needed to know about. Begrudgingly, I said, "Yes, we will do an autopsy." I almost immediately regretted that decision.

As we entered the chapel to see Noble again, I noticed that his head shape was completely different because of the autopsy. He didn't look like the perfect, round child that I said goodbye to a few days prior. Crossing my arms, I walked away in anger. I sat in a chair far away from my once perfect child stating in anger, "He doesn't look the same. It's not Noble." I felt waves of nausea and regret hit my stomach and heart. I should have stuck to my gut reaction when they asked me to do an autopsy and said, "No, I don't want an autopsy." Now, my perfect child was marred forever and it was my fault.

I left the church to get some fresh air. My mom followed me to make sure that I was okay. "It doesn't look like Noble," I continued. "I don't want to see him like that or remember him like that." My mom tried to comfort me, but I was inconsolable. We never had to make decisions like this before. We were out of our minds with grief, struggling to string together a logical thought process after Noble died, much less knowing whether or not we should donate his organs or do an autopsy.

After attempting to process the regret of my decision, we headed back into the funeral parlor to meet with the director and plan the details of the funeral. Surprisingly calm, I made decisions with ease and signed the paperwork. Did we want to do a luncheon afterwards? We left that undecided and made a plan to go to a restaurant with close friends and family members after the funeral if we felt up for it. Leaving the room after the meeting, I stopped dead in my tracks letting out an earth-shattering wail while my entire body quaked with grief. Sobbing and travailing in pain, my parents and husband all rushed over to comfort me. Crying themselves, everyone felt helpless at the enormity of my grief while the funeral director said, "It shouldn't be like this, I am so sorry."

I vividly remember those moments of spontaneous eruption of grief from my body. I remember grieving loud and almost out of body, my whole body shaking. And I remember grieving openly, in public, giving myself permission to feel and to be vulnerable in front of family, friends, strangers and neighbors.

Looking back, I wonder how strange that time was. I intuitively knew what I needed to grieve and to heal. We kept Noble Thomas with us for 24-hours after his death in the hospital. My husband gave Noble a bath, rubbing his entire body with lavender, singing over him and preparing him for burial. We had brought the lavender soap and lavender essential oil to give Noble his first bath in the hospital after he was born. Instead, the lavender soap and essential oil became a symbol of loss up until today.

During our process of grieving, we noticed that some people were comfortable with our open manner of grieving whereas others didn't know how to respond to our deep, intense emotions. In general, Western culture is not comfortable with open grieving and grieving in a communal manner. In fact, in the U.S., there has been a history of the privatization of grief. Many people who lose loved ones grieve in solitude, without community support before and after the funeral of a loved one.

Could it be that people don't know how to offer support and love after the loss of a loved one or that people don't want to say or do the wrong thing? Or could it be that without strong cultural grieving rituals, we are lost to know what to do as a community? Or are we "too busy" to grieve?

Some people point to the Plague as a time when grieving rituals began to be discarded.[1] So many people died during the Plague that there wasn't enough time or energy to perform the normal grieving rituals. Further, people did not understand what caused the plague and they didn't want to perform any bathing rituals out of fear that they would contract the plague themselves. Prior to this time, it was common practice for loves ones who were grieving to bathe the deceased and prepare their body for burial. This was a common grieving ritual in the Western culture that has been lost.

Another belief surrounding why we have lost our grieving rituals is that our culture is obsessed with living forever and focused around prolonging life. People in the Western culture tend to avoid the topic of death and live in denial to the reality of death. Other cultures around the world embrace death as part of living and have strong beliefs about life after death that allow them to feel more comfortable with the concept of death. As a culture, we are obsessed with not dying, with preserving life out of the fear of death. Thus, many people in our culture do not develop a belief system surrounding what happens after we die and manage to avoid the topic altogether.

Further, does the lack of grieving rituals in our culture set the stage for an inability to properly grieve and recover after the loss of a loved one? And does an inability to grieve allow for an opportunity for mental illness to develop? Many non-Western cultures have maintained grieving rituals and death ceremonies, allowing for long-term grief, making death a part of life and placing communal support around the family who is actively grieving.

In South Africa, where my husband is from, the body of the deceased is washed and prepared for the wake, which happens in the home of the family. For one full day, family, friends and the neighboring community pour into the home to say goodbye and see the open casket of the deceased. The next day, the funeral occurs for another full day. Everyone stops working for at least 2 days to grieve and support one another. For weeks and even months after the death of the loved one, neighbors, friends and family bring food and care for the family who is grieving.

When we planned the funeral for Noble, I was adamant to have an open casket. I wanted everyone to meet Noble because of how beautiful he was. I also felt that I needed an open casket in order to say goodbye properly. I felt that it was important for everyone to tangibly connect with his life and his death in order to heal and grieve. I did receive some feedback from family members who thought that the casket should be closed. I dismissed their opinions because of my strong sense that an open casket would be more healing for me and for those who came to the funeral.

When we lost Noble Thomas, my husband and I set up visiting hours for family, friends and neighbors similar to the custom in South Africa. We shared Noble's story and the pictures that were taken of Noble while we were in the hospital with him. Also, 3 days after Noble died, we held a prayer vigil for close family and friends to sing, grieve and pray with us. I cried during the entire prayer vigil, for about 2 hours straight, but at the end, I felt relief and the beginning seed of peace.

Grieving out loud, in front of our family, friends, neighbors and community brought healing, love and peace to our hearts. The death of my son was not the first death that I had to process; in fact, I have become increasingly more comfortable with the concept of death because of my work with late stage cancer patients. I daily interact with clients who may or may not survive their diagnosis. I consider it a privilege to walk with someone through a cancer diagnosis and to explore concepts surrounding life and death, spiritual connection, healing and preparation for life or for death.

In his research, David Spiegel found that being able to express emotions like anger and grief can improve survival rates in cancer.[2] I often think about what it would feel like to still carry the trauma, emotional pain and weight of the loss of Noble in my body. I believe that many people still carry trauma and grief in their soul and body as a result of not being able to grieve fully the loss of a loved one. Some remain in denial, some lack the communal support in the grieving process and others struggle to grieve because of their beliefs or because of a complicated situation of loss. Some people may lack the emotional intelligence or the innate ability to release deep emotions of grief. Some people have certain beliefs or even unsolidified beliefs about death that may complicate the grieving process. Some people carry the fear of death with them into grieving and this can hinder the grieving process as well.

How comfortable are you with the concept of death? Do you have solidified beliefs about what happens after we die? Do you have situations of loss that you have struggled to grieve and process fully? Let's explore this concept further to help you examine your beliefs about death or to help you find beliefs surrounding death. If you don't feel ready to die, if you don't feel peace-surrounding death or if you are facing a life-threatening illness like cancer and you want to prepare yourself for death, you may find this section invaluable. **The sooner that we can come to terms with the reality that we all have an incurable disease: death, the sooner that we can accept death as a part of living.**

I remember when the first person close to me died, my grandma. I can picture the funeral, walking by the open casket and sobbing not only for the loss of my grandma, but also for the finality of death. I was young, only 15-16 years old, and I hadn't explored the concept of death; thus, my beliefs surrounding death were not solidified.

My grandma had developed Alzheimer's disease several years prior and progressively lost her memory each time we went to see her. One day, my grandma looked at us with a blank stare and began talking about her daughter that lives in Lake Elmo right in front of my mom, her daughter. That moment was so painful as it felt like we had already lost her. I was close with my grandma; we had one night a month where each of the grandkids could sleep at grandma and grandpa's house by themselves. I would make cookies with grandma, go to the library with her and play with my favorite marble game in the attic. I would stare in awe at all of the musical instruments in my grandpa's den. He was an avid musician and could play by ear. I can still smell the aroma of my grandpa smoking a pipe in his den, as he often would while listening to his favorite jazz music.

When my grandma died, it felt like the loss of a loved one compounded with the loss of innocence surrounding the illusion of immortality. For the first time in my life, I had to face not only the death of my beloved grandma, but also death as a concept that I would face over and over again until my own impending death. This concept was horrifying and triggered a deep sense of confusion and sadness in its own right. I had no solid beliefs about life after death, just a vague sense of heaven without any strong convictions or spiritual experiences to confirm the possibility of experiencing a better place after death.

At the time of my grandma's death, I was preparing to go to college and start life as a real adult. In a couple of years, I was going to move out of the safety and comfort of my childhood home. It was also around the time that I got caught shoplifting and when I noticed the unsettling feelings of emptiness and a lack of purpose in my life.

When I went to college after losing my grandma, I started to have panic attacks every night. At first, I didn't know what it was. After having panic attacks a few times, I figured out what was happening. I started to find strategies that would help like talking to a friend prior to going to bed at night to unravel my overwhelming thoughts.

At that time, I started yearning for peace. Our human spirit longs for peace and alignment with our true sense of self. In my first semester at college, I was confused and lost in my understanding of the world and spirituality. But, I was also determined and willing to seek spiritual understanding until I found what it was I was searching for.

It is strange to search for something that you don't know yet and that seems to escape you like a vapor. I had shadows of understanding the next step to take, but it was not clear at the time the direction I was heading. However, I knew that I was on a path of spiritual discovery. You may feel right now that you are on a path of spiritual discovery and that you are open to whatever spiritual connection needed to bring comfort, peace and clarity. My prayer for you is that you would find the spiritual connection that you seek.

When we feel uncomfortable with a funeral or the aging process in general, we may not have solidified our spiritual beliefs. Do you notice feeling uncomfortable with the concept of aging and death? It is common in the Western world to avoid topics of aging and death because of the uncertainty and uncomfortable feelings involved. Many people carry negative views on aging and attempt to reverse signs of aging through dying their hair or buying lotions to remove wrinkles.

Our beliefs about aging have a powerful impact upon our biology. In fact, researchers have found that negative views of aging can put you at risk for developing Alzheimer's disease or experiencing an earlier death.[3] Researchers Ellen Langer at Harvard University and Becca Levy at Yale School of Public Health found that having positive views about aging improves your health and extends your life more than exercising or quitting smoking![4]

How can we change our mindset and outlook on aging? I know that I find myself more confident, more comfortable in my own skin and bolder in the expression of my unique identity as I age. I think that we would all benefit from finding more positives than negatives in aging and embrace this beautiful process called life!

As we continue to explore how beliefs intersect with our biology, it is helpful to understand the following terms: the nocebo effect and the placebo effect. The placebo effect is the expectation or belief a patient has in a good outcome with a treatment and how this belief can positively impact the body's response to that particular protocol. The nocebo effect is the exact opposite of the placebo effect and the term nocebo literally means, "to harm." The nocebo effect is an expectation surrounding negative treatment outcomes and how a negative belief about a prognosis can lead to a decline in health.

The power of the placebo and nocebo effect can be quite literally life or death. For example, in the 1970s, a Nashville physician Clifton Meador diagnosed Sam Londe with cancer of the esophagus. Doctor Meador told Sam that esophageal cancer was fatal 100% of the time. Everyone around Sam Londe believed that he would die, including Sam. A few weeks after his diagnosis, Sam Lunde died as expected. However, the autopsy found very little cancer in his body.[5] In fact, there was no trace of esophageal cancer only a few spots on his lung and in his liver. Sam died with cancer, but not because of cancer. Did he die because he believed the prognosis from his doctor and the nocebo effect had a pronounced impact on his biology?

More recently, an individual involved in a clinical trial for antidepressants "overdosed" by taking 29 capsules. He was admitted to the hospital for many symptoms including hypotension. When he found out that he was taking the placebo capsule, the "symptoms" of overdosing completely disappeared.[6]

To highlight the power of the placebo effect, let's look at a study published in the New England Journal of Medicine. Dr. Bruce Moseley at The Baylor School of Medicine performed a study on knee surgery.[7] He wanted to discover which surgical approach was more effective for his patients. He prepared 3 groups of patients for knee surgery, including the placebo control group. The placebo control group did not have surgery, but participants were prepared for surgery just like the other 2 groups in the study. In fact, the placebo control group did not find out that they did not have surgery until 2 years after the study.

Surprisingly to everyone, including Dr. Bruce Moseley, the placebo control group showed just as much improvement as the 2 groups of participants that actually had surgery. In fact, one particular participant was walking with a cane prior to the study and afterwards, he could play basketball with his grandkids. He was a part of the placebo control group and did not go through actual surgery. Two years after the study, he was shocked to find out that his improvement was entirely based upon the placebo effect!

What fosters the development of the placebo effect in a cancer patient? According to Evers, a health psychologist at the University of Leiden, warmth, empathy and trust between a patient and his or her practitioner enhances the placebo effect and reduces the nocebo effect.[8] What magnifies the nocebo effect? A lack of trust, a lack of empathy, a lack of connection and warmth between a health practitioner and his or her patient will increase the nocebo effect and decrease the placebo effect. Make sure that you feel warmth, empathy and trust between you and your health practitioners during a cancer diagnosis in order to enhance the placebo effect and diminish the nocebo effect.

When a cancer diagnosis occurs, our beliefs surrounding our body's ability to heal need to be reexamined. It is important to challenge any negative beliefs regarding cancer and death, even when those beliefs come from your oncologist. It is critical to build the belief factor that your body is wired to heal given the right support and the right approach.

Perfectionism & Spirituality

We all have a longing for something greater than us and for something more perfect than us. I had been a recovering perfectionist for many years when I discovered the gift of my imperfections. I will end this book with my story of overcoming perfectionism and healing from an incurable disease.

When I was 17 years old, I was diagnosed with PCOS, Polycystic Ovary Syndrome. I was told that I might never be able to have children because of the cysts on my ovaries. I was given a medication to take for the rest of my life along with no hope for healing. According to my doctor, PCOS was an incurable disease.

I lived with this diagnosis for many years and struggled to accept my fate of having an incurable disease that would hinder my ability to mother my own children. After I began to make a spiritual connection in my life, I began to question my prognosis.

Eight months prior to my commitment to work at a non-profit in Cape Town, I decided to go off of my medication to pursue healing from PCOS. I started to work with a chiropractor and an herbalist to deal with the root causes of the cysts on my ovaries. However, nothing seemed to heal the root causes of the cystic condition, as my symptoms only got worse.

Prior to leaving for Cape Town, I gave up trying to find the solution to my incurable disease. I had tried, but failed to heal myself. Besides, I was leaving for a new adventure and I was focused on all of the details of my trip. Arriving in South Africa, I began my work at the orphanage and the high school for at-risk youth. I was overwhelmed by the needs around me as I had never faced systemic poverty and all of the challenges surrounding poverty: trauma, abuse, neglect, drug abuse, addiction, gang activity, hopelessness, teenage pregnancy, HIV/AIDS and more.

Prior to living in South Africa, I had achieved a lot and felt like I had a lot to offer the world. However, when you are surrounded by the depth of vulnerability and need in situations of systemic poverty, you begin to question your ability to impact the world. I started to struggle with deep feelings of guilt and inadequacy.

Beyond the guilt that I felt, I sensed a heavy weight of condemnation, that I was not good enough and that there was something inherently wrong with me. I found a YouTube teaching online that shared more information about the root causes and psychology surrounding condemnation. The teacher on the video said the following, "The deeper root of anxiety and fear is condemnation, the sense that you are not good enough and that you are rejected." His teaching continued and all that he was saying was resonating deep within me. He was speaking my language and exposing the deeper roots of my perpetual struggle with anxiety.

He spoke about perfectionism as well and how we can strive to get everything perfect and right, but we always seem to miss the mark of perfection. "Do you ever feel like you have a voice in your head like a stern teacher telling you all of the things that you are doing wrong? That is the voice of condemnation." The man continued to speak, his words echoing into the deepest chambers of my being.

The voice of condemnation that he spoke about was very familiar to me. I heard the voice of condemnation after a conversation with a teacher at the school in Cape Town saying, "You should have said it that way or communicated this, now she is going to think this awful thing about you or she is going to do the wrong thing and it's all going to be your fault." I heard the voice of condemnation talking to me when I held my baby, Anam, saying, "You are not doing her any good. In fact, you are only going to further traumatize her when you leave the country."

I was a perfectionist at heart and ever since I was a young child, I strived to achieve and accomplish perfection in every area of my life. However, when I would try to be perfect in school, my physical health would fail and I would start to gain weight and not take care of my body properly. When I would start to focus on my physical health, start running and eating healthy, my grades began to slip. When I would focus on my grades again, my relationships would begin to be distant and I would feel isolated and alone. Then, I would try to find balance again by focusing on my relationships and everything else would fall apart.

The voice of condemnation was always questioning me, what I said, what I did, telling me how I was failing in life. Until this YouTube teaching exposed the voice of condemnation to me, making my internal battle clear and apparent. **The teacher went on to say something that changed my life forever, "When you strive for perfection and fall short, you may find yourself under the voice of condemnation. At this point, simply reach out to perfection. Jesus lived the perfect life that you cannot live and if you receive from him the gift of righteousness, you will be set free from the voice of condemnation."** When I heard those words, I believed them. Next, I felt something significant happen to my body; I literally felt a weight lift off of my shoulders. All of a sudden, I felt light, like I was floating in the air. My mind became quiet and the voice of condemnation disappeared. I felt space in my mind that I didn't have before along with a calming, spiritual presence.

On top of it all, the next day, I was healed of PCOS. Ten years previously, I had been diagnosed with an incurable disease and all of my symptoms left within 24-hours of a profound, internal transformation. The deeper root of my cystic condition was condemnation, not an iodine deficiency like I had thought.

When I received that seed of perfection through the life of Jesus, I became peaceful about dying, believing that the seed of perfection would be accepted one day when I died and that I could enter into the perfection of heaven forever. The puzzle pieces of spirituality began to fit together for me and I felt like I could now manage the reality of life along with the reality of death.

Bronnie Ware, a palliative care nurse in Australia, discovered that the common regret of those dying is the following: people who are dying wish that they had the courage to live a life true to themselves and not the life that others expected of them.[9] When you are facing a near-death disease, you have the opportunity to receive more clarity on what matters most and what matters least in life. Many times, my clients with cancer rearrange their lives in order to live out their true identity and passions instead of pleasing people.

Cancer can be a gift for those who would receive it in that manner. Cancer can expose dead areas in your life to allow you to come alive in ways that you were too fearful of prior to your diagnosis. My hope and prayer is that cancer will lead you into your best life yet, to the truest sense of your identity. I also hope that you find a deep spiritual connection that would ground you in eternal hope, peace and comfort.

One of my clients, Savanna, is a perfect example of what we have been discussing throughout this section. Savanna grew up in a large family with a lot of siblings. She was the youngest and the smallest of her siblings. She remembers being overlooked and misunderstood a lot growing up. She also remembers interactions with her father that left her feeling not important and not loved. In one of our sessions, the following came up for her, "I always wanted to feel loved by my dad, but I would leave interactions with him unsure of where I stood with him. One specific event occurred when I was young, 5 or 6 years old, I was sitting on his lap looking at a catalogue with him. I pointed out a few things that I wanted and my dad criticized me by saying, "How can you say something so foolish? We aren't getting any of them." He promptly took me off of his lap and sat me on the ground while expressing anger towards me. I ended up feeling confused, ashamed and embarrassed. This is one of many examples where I left an interaction with my dad feeling unloved and confused.

My parents worried out loud while I grew up and were generally negative people. I lived with constant knots of anxiety in my stomach and learned to 'wait for the next shoe to drop' as it seemed like problems magnified constantly in my family. There was palpable fear in my home because of the expectation of the next bad thing to happen. Basically, I lived with a sense of impending doom, fear and anxiety.

Another time that I felt misunderstood was when my sister came home from school and declared to me, 'You are narcissistic.' She had learned that word in school that day. I didn't know what she meant when she said that, but I was devastated. I felt like I was inherently wrong and screwed up, but I didn't know what to do about it.

When I became a mom myself, I did my best, but I have regrets and felt like I didn't do all that I wanted to do for my children. I try to connect with my children, but many times I feel like my husband is the favorite and I'm second best. Whenever our children come over even as adults to bring something for my husband and not for me, I feel like I'm not good enough and that they don't love me the way that they love their dad. All of this stems from how I grew up and feeling like I wasn't loveable."

We had been working together for about 6 months before receiving the results of her cancer blood work. She had been diagnosed with Stage IV Multiple Myeloma (MM) a few months before we started working together. The recommendation from her oncologist was palliative chemotherapy. When Savanna and I first started working together, she told me the following, "My oncologist told me that I need to be on chemotherapy for the rest of my life and I don't really know what that means." We discussed the difference between palliative treatments and curative treatments. Savanna was devastated when she discovered that she was on palliative treatments. She also felt horrible on chemotherapy and lived with many side effects. She had done 13 rounds of chemotherapy up until that point and her cancer blood markers were starting to get worse. The chemotherapy wasn't working. Savanna decided to stop palliative chemotherapy treatments while pursuing a second opinion at a leading cancer research hospital near her home.

In the meantime, Savanna began working with Cancer Peace University and two other integrative doctors to support her holistically. After 6 months, her cancer blood work had gone up from 4.5 to 5.7. She called me one day after receiving her results, crying incessantly. She cried in desperation while asking me,

"Do any of your clients experience cancer blood markers getting worse before they improve or does this mean that I'm going to die?" My heart paining for Savanna, I responded softly, "No, Savanna, this doesn't mean you're going to die. Numbers can go up and down in a journey of healing, but this doesn't mean anything definitive. It just means that we need to explore what other support your body needs and look at what we might be missing on the emotional side."

At this point, we had redesigned a lot of memories from Savanna's childhood; she had forgiven herself and others while diminishing a perpetual sense of anxiety. In fact, in the beginning of working together, Savanna called me every day in a panic. We would talk through how she was feeling, she would get direction on what to do next and then she would feel better. I knew we were making progress on the emotional side when I stopped getting phone calls every day from Savanna.

However, after 6 months of working together and finding that her cancer numbers had not improved yet, I knew we were missing something on the emotional side. I asked Savanna, "What is still lingering for you emotionally?" Savanna responded to me, "I still feel this sense of impending doom, like the other shoe is about to drop." I considered her words before responding, "OK, I think you may be dealing with the voice of condemnation. Let's talk this through. Are you hard on yourself? Do you question everything you say and do?" Savanna responded immediately, "Yes, especially with my children. Every time I reach out to my children and wait for their response, I think, oh, I should have said this or did this. I just don't always know how to reach out to them and connect emotionally. I am a deep feeler and I cry a lot, but my children don't like emotions. My children don't like when I cry in front of them, so I don't know how to express myself around them."

I continued saying, "I think that you are dealing with condemnation. Condemnation is a general sense of not measuring up to an ideal standard of being. It is the sense that you will be rejected if people knew everything about you. Condemnation is the voice in your head that always tells you where you are missing it, where you messed up and where you will probably mess up in the future. It is the voice pushing you to strive to be perfect or to seem perfect to those around you. It is the voice that wants you to hide yourself, your imperfections and perform for people around you. You don't have to live like that. Jesus lived the perfect life that you cannot live and you can receive the gift of righteousness that begins the process of perfecting you.

When I was in Cape Town many years ago, I was dealing with guilt and condemnation like you are now. I felt like nothing I did or said would ever be good enough and that I would never make the impact I wanted to make on the world as a result. I felt this heavy weight of condemnation on my shoulders. Then, I watched a video that changed my life. The teacher on the video said, 'The deeper root of anxiety and fear is condemnation. Jesus lived the perfect life that you can never live, but you can receive perfection and the gift of grace that will bring spiritual freedom, connection and healing to your body.' I believed that his words were true and at that moment, I felt something heavy break off of my shoulders. I felt like I was floating. The next day, I was healed of my incurable disease, PCOS, and my mind was freed from the voice of condemnation. Do you want to receive this gift of grace from Jesus to free you now?"

Savanna responded, "Yes, I do." I prayed a short prayer and then I waited as Savanna received the spiritual impact of the prayer. I waited for quite a while. Two minutes passed and I asked Savanna softly, "Are you noticing anything?" She didn't respond. I thought, that's weird, but I kept waiting to see if she was still there. A minute passed and all of a sudden, Savanna spoke, "I'm still here! After you prayed, I fell onto my bed and felt a tingling feeling run throughout my whole body. I wasn't afraid and I felt like I was floating. But, I couldn't speak. I was lying on my bed, trying to respond to you, but nothing would come out of my mouth. I feel so light and free! Thank you, Thank you, Thank you!" I was thrilled that Savanna had the same experience as me.

The other amazing part of Savanna's story is that a few weeks later, her cancer blood work improved dramatically. This time, her cancer blood work numbers drawn by her oncologist went down from 5.7 to 1.69, 0.05 away from the normal range. A few weeks later, another blood draw happened through her oncologist and this time, her numbers moved down to 1.4416, in the normal range for the first time after her diagnosis! Her oncologist declared that she was now in remission!

Now, I want to ask you, do you also deal with a heavy weight of condemnation and guilt, feeling like you are missing the mark in some areas of your life? Have you tried to change and perfect yourself, but feel like you have come up short? **Would you like to be free from the weight of condemnation?** If you resonate with my story and Savanna's experience, I want you to say this short prayer with me and follow the questions in the workbook afterwards, "God, I don't know what I believe about the spiritual realm fully, but I want to connect spiritually in an authentic way. I have felt like I have missed the mark in some areas of my life and I'm not measuring up to my ideal self. **I know that I am not perfect and that I have made mistakes and haven't always done the right thing. Can you set me free from condemnation and give me the gift of righteousness through Jesus? Thank you for setting me free."** Now, wait and take a deep breath while you receive from the spiritual realm what you need to be free and relationally connected to God. How do you feel? Continue this process with me in the companion workbook.

What a journey! Thank you so much for following me through this journey of pursuing a profound, internal transformation. We have made it to the pinnacle and it is our hope at Cancer Peace University that you have experienced a profound, internal transformation yourself! We also hope that this transformation has impacted your biology like some of the client stories we have shared in this book.

During the storm of your cancer diagnosis, we also hope that you have experienced collateral beauty out of an experience that you may never have chosen for yourself, but that has an opportunity to profoundly change your life for the better. Our Cancer Peace University community is here for you to support you, guide you and help you find the inspiration and hope that countless others have found throughout a cancer diagnosis. Know this: you are not alone and we are here to celebrate your victories and mourn your disappointments with you. **Never give into fear or give up hope that the path of spontaneous remission is laid out before you. Further, it is up to you to walk courageously into the storm of your diagnosis to discover pieces of the puzzle of your identity and purpose on earth and to find peace with your own mortality. This is the gift of cancer that we hope you find.**

References

Preface:

1. Moritz, Andreas. (2009). *Cancer Is Not a Disease, It's A Survival Mechanism.* Third Edition. United States of America: Ener-Chi Wellness Press. Page 116.

Section 1: Getting Right with Me
Chapter 1: A Change of Mind

1. Carreira, Helena; Williams, Rachael; Muller, Martin; Harewood, Rhea; Stanway, Susannah; Bhaskaran, Krishnan. **Associations Between Breast Cancer Survivorship & Adverse Mental Health Outcomes: A Systematic Review.** *JNCI: Journal of The National Cancer Institute,* Volume 110, Issue 12, December 2018, Pages 1311-1327: 07 November 2018: https://academic.oup.com/jnci/article/110/12/1311/5164 282)
2. Neff, K. (2011). *Self-compassion: Stop beating yourself up and leave insecurity behind.* New York: William Morrow.
3. Sissa Medialab, "The Good Side of the Prion: A Molecule That Is Not Only Dangerous, but Can Help the Brain Grow," *Science Daily,* February 14, 2013, https://www.sciencedaily.com/releases/2013/02/130214 075437.htm
4. Eric R. Kandel, *In Search of Memory: The Emergence of a New Science of Mind (*New York: Norton, 2006).
5. Church, Dawson. (2008). *The Genie in Your Genes.* Fulton, CA: Energy Psychology Press. Pg. 65.; "Epigenetics: A Web Tour," *Science, https://www.sciencemag.org/site/feature/plus/sfg/resear ch/rsch_epigenetics.xhtml;* Ethan Watters, "DNA Is Not Destiny: The New Science of Epigenetics Rewrites the

Rules of Disease, Heredity, and Identity," *Discover,* November 2006, http://discovermagazine.com/2006/nov/cover.

6. Elizabeth Pennisi, "Behind the Scenes of Gene Expression," *Science* 293, no. 553 (2001): 1064-67.

7. Church, Dawson. (2008). *The Genie in Your Genes.* Fulton, CA: Energy Psychology Press. Pg. 65. "Local and Nonlocal Effects of Coherent Heart Frequencies on Conformational Changes of DNA." https://appreciativeinquiry.champlain.edu/wp-content/uploads/2016/01/HeartMath-article.pdf. https://www.brianlukeseaward.com/downloads/SuperStress-WELCOA-Seaward.pdf. "Cancer Statistics and Views of Causes," *Science News* 115, no. 2 (January 13, 1979): 23; H.F. Nijhout "Metaphors and the Role of Genes and Development," *BioEssays* 12 (1990): 444-46; W. C. Willett, "Balancing Lifestyle and Genomics Research for Disease Prevention," *Science* 296 (2002): 695-98; C. B. Pert, *Molecules of Emotion: Why You Feel The Way You Feel* (New York: Simon and Schuster, 1997); B. Lipton, *The Biology of Belief: Unleashing the Power of Consciousness, Matter and Miracles* (Santa Cruz, CA: Mountain of Love Productions, 2008).

8. Glen Rein and Rollin McCarty, "Local and Nonlocal Effects of Coherent Heart Frequencies on Conformational Changes of DNA," Proceedings of the Joint USPA/IAPR Psychotronics Conference, Milwaukee, Wisconsin, 1993, https://www.heartmath.org/articles-of-the-heart/personal-development/you-can-change-your-dna/; Rollin, McCraty et al., "Modulation of DNA Conformation By Heart-focused Intention." HeartMath Research Center, Institute of HeartMath, Publications no. 03-08, Boulder Creek, CA, 2003.

Section 1: Getting Right With Me
Chapter 2: Releasing Regret & Shame

1. Pennebaker, J. W., Kiecolt-Glaser, J., and Glaser, R. (1988). Disclosure of traumas and immune function: Health Implications for psychotherapy. *Journal of Consulting and Clinical Psychology, 56:* 239-245.
2. Petrie, K. J., Booth, R. J., and Pennebaker, J. W. (1998). The immunological effects of thought suppression. *Journal of Personality and Social Psychology, 75:* 1264-1272.
3. Brown, Brene. (2012). *Daring Greatly: How the Courage to Be Vulnerable Transforms the Way We Live, Love, Parent, and Lead.* New York: Penguin Random House. Pg. 117-130.
4. Pennebaker, J.W. (2004). *Writing to heal: A guided journal for recovering from trauma and emotional upheaval.* Oakland: New Harbinger Publications.

Section 1: Getting Right with Me
Chapter 3: Freeing Your Mind from Imprints of Trauma

1. https://pubmed.ncbi.nlm.nih.gov/31104722/; "Dr. Vincent Felitti: Reflections on the Adverse Childhood Experiences (ACE) Study," YouTube video, 32:33, posted by National Congress of American Indians, June 23, 2016, https://www.youtube.com/watch?v=-ns8ko9-ljU
2. Marcus E. Raichle et al., "A Default Mode of Brain Function: A Brief History of an Evolving Idea" *Neuroimage* 37 (2007): 1083-90.
3. G. Vijuk and A. S. Coates, "Survival of patients with visceral metastatic melanoma from an occult primary lesion: a retrospective matched cohort study," *Annals of Oncology,* vol. 9, no. 4, (1998): 419-422.

4. Richard J. Davidson et al., "Alterations in Brain and Immune Function Produced by Mindfulness Meditation," *Psychosomatic Medicine 65* (2003): 564-70.
5. Marcus E. Raichle, "The Brain's Dark Energy," *Scientific American,* March 20, 2012, 44-49, https://science.sciencemag.org/content/314/5803/1249.full; Raichle et al., "A Default Mode of Brain Function," 1083-90.
6. Yvette I. Sheline et al., "The Default Mode Network and Self-Referential Processes in Depression," *Proceedings of the National Academy of Sciences USA 106,* no.6 (January 26, 2009): 1942-47.
7. Brier et al., "Loss of Intranetwork and Internetwork Resting State Functional Connections with Alzheimer's Disease Progression."
8. J. Paul Hamilton et al., "Default Mode and Task Positive Network Activity in Major Depressive Disorder: Implications for Adaptive and Maladaptive Rumination," *Biological Psychiatry 70,* no. 4 (2011): 327-33.
9. Caroline M. Leaf, "Mind Mapping: A Therapeutic Technique for Closed Head Injury," unpublished master's dissertation (University of Pretoria, Pretoria, South Africa), 1990.

Section 1: Getting Right With Me
Chapter 4: Embracing Your Eccentricity

1. https://www.psychologytoday.com/us/blog/psychiatry-the-people/201811/the-hippocampus-self-esteem-and-physical-health
2. M.G. Marmot, S. Stansfeld, C. Patel, F. North, J. Head, I. White, E. Brunner, A. Feeney, M.G. Marmot, G. Davey Smith. "Health inequalities among British civil servants: the Whitehall II study." *The Lancet, Volume*

337, Issue 8754 (1991): 1387-1393, ISSN 0140-6736. https://www.sciencedirect.com/science/article/abs/pii/01 4067369193068K; https://www.bmj.com/content/314/7080/558

3. Shealy, Norman. (2005). *Life Beyond 100: Secrets of the Fountain of Youth.* First Edition. Tarcher.

4. Carroll, Barbara. (2012). *Healing the Cancer Personality.* First Edition. Life Application Ministries Publications; http://www.alternative-cancer-care.com/AlternativeCancerTreatment.html

5. Grano, Niklas. "Impulsivity, health-related behaviour and disease: A prospective study." UNIVERSITY OF HELSINKI Department of Psychology Studies 48: 2008; https://helda.helsinki.fi/bitstream/handle/10138/19862/i mpulsiv.pdf?sequence=1

6. Mucci Nicola, Giorgi Gabriele, De Pasquale Ceratti Stefano, Fiz-Pérez Javier, Mucci Federico, Arcangeli Giulio. "Anxiety, Stress-Related Factors, and Blood Pressure in Young Adults." *Frontiers in Psychology*, Volume 7 (2016): 1682, ISSN 1664-1078 https://www.frontiersin.org/articles/10.3389/fpsyg.2016. 01682/full#B74; Pan Y, Cai W, Cheng Q, Dong W, An T, Wang J. "Association between anxiety and hypertension: a systematic review and meta-analysis of epidemiological studies." *Neuropsychiatr Dis Treat.* 2015; 11:1121-1130 https://doi.org/10.2147/NDT.S77710 https://www.dovepress.com/association-between-anxiety-and-hypertension-a-systematic-review-and-m-peer-reviewed-article-NDT; https://www.dailymail.co.uk/health/article-1028864/Your-personality-type-decide-makes-ill.html

7. Carroll, Barbara. (2012). *Healing The Cancer Personality.* First Edition. Life Application Ministries

Publications; https://www.dailymail.co.uk/health/article-1028864/Your-personality-type-decide-makes-ill.html
8. Jean-Philippe Gouin, Janice K. Kiecolt-Glaser, William B. Malarkey, Ronald Glaser. "The influence of anger expression on wound healing." *Brain, Behavior, and Immunity,* Volume 22, Issue 5 (2008): 699-708, ISSN 0889-1591; https://www.sciencedirect.com/science/article/abs/pii/S0889159107002644
9. Levy, Becca, Slade, Martin, Kasl, and Stanislav. "Longevity Increased by Positive Self-Perceptions of Aging." *Journal of Personality & Social Psychology,* Volume 83 (2002); https://www.researchgate.net/publication/11232977_Longevity_Increased_by_Positive_Self-Perceptions_of_Aging
10. Segerstrom, S. C., Taylor, S. E., Kemeny, M. E., & Fahey, J. L. Optimism is associated with mood, coping, and immune change in response to stress. *Journal of Personality and Social Psychology, 74*(6) (1998): 1646–1655; https://psycnet.apa.org/record/1998-02892-019
11. Leshan, Lawrence. (1994). *Cancer As A Turning Point: A Handbook for Those with Cancer, their Families and Health Professionals.* Revised Edition. Plume.
12. Mate, Gabor M.D. (2011). *When The Body Says No: Exploring The Stress-Disease Connection.* Canada: Vintage; https://www.alive.com/health/the-cancer-personality/
13. Temoshok, Lydia. Kneier, Andrew W. "Repressive coping reactions in patients with malignant melanoma as compared to cardiovascular disease patients." *Journal of Psychosomatic Research,* Volume 28, Issue 2 (1984): 145-155, ISSN 0022-3999, *https://www.sciencedirect.com/science/article/abs/pii/0022399984900084*

14. Kune GA, Kune S, Watson LF, Bahnson CB. "Personality as a risk factor in large bowel cancer: data from the Melbourne Colorectal Cancer Study." *Psychol Med,* Feb; 21, 1 (1991): 29-41; *https://pubmed.ncbi.nlm.nih.gov/2047503/*
15. Pert, Candace B. (2003). *Molecules Of Emotion: The Science Behind Mind-Body Medicine.* New York: Scribner.

Section 1: Getting Right With Me
Chapter 5: Digging Deeper

1. A. J. Cunningham, C. V. Edmonds, C. Phillips, et al., "A Randomized Controlled Trial of the Effects on Survival of Group Psychological Therapy for Women with Metastatic Breast Cancer," *Psycho-Oncology 7,* no. 6 (1998): 508-517.
2. A. J. Cunningham, C. Phillips, J. Stephen, C. Edmonds, "Fighting for life: a qualitative analysis of the process of psychotherapy-assisted self-help in patients with metastatic cancer," *Integrative Cancer Therapies 1,* no. 2 (2002). 146-161.
3. Pennebaker JW. "Expressive Writing in Psychological Science." *Perspectives on Psychological Science.* Volume 13, Issue 2 (2018): 226-229; https://journals.sagepub.com/doi/10.1177/17456916177 07315

Section 2: Relationships Reflect Me: What Do You See?
Chapter 1: The Broken Heart

1. Karin Brulliard, "A Woman's Dog Died, and Doctors Say It Literally Broke Her Heart," Washington Post, October 19, 2017; www.washingtonpost.com/news/animalia/wp/2017/10/1

    9/a-womans-dog-died-and-doctors-say-her-heart-literally-broke/

2. https://health.clevelandclinic.org/how-coronavirus-is-causing-broken-heart-syndrome/

3. Cramer MJ, De Boeck B, Melman PG, Sieswerda GJ. "The 'broken heart' syndrome: What can be learned from the tears and distress?" *Neth Heart J.* Volume 15, Issue 9 (2007): 283-5; https://www.ncbi.nlm.nih.gov/pmc/articles/PMC1995104/

4. Wittstein HS, Thiemann DR, Lima JAC, Baughman KL, Schulman SP, Gerstenblith G, et al. Neurohumoral features of myocardial stunning due to sudden emotional stress. New Engl J Med 2005; 352:539-48.

5. Ethan Kross, Marc G. Berman, Walter Mischel, Edward E. Smith, Tor D. Wager. "Social rejection shares somatosensory representations with physical pain." *Proceedings of the National Academy of Sciences Apr* 2011, 108 (15) 6270-6275; https://www.pnas.org/content/108/15/6270.long

6. Pert, Candace B. (2003). *Molecules Of Emotion: The Science Behind Mind-Body Medicine.* New York: Scribner; Temoshok, Lydia. Kneier, Andrew W. "Repressive coping reactions in patients with malignant melanoma as compared to cardiovascular disease patients." *Journal of Psychosomatic Research,* Volume 28, Issue 2 (1984): 145-155, ISSN 0022-3999; *https://www.sciencedirect.com/science/article/abs/pii/0022399984900084*

7. Adams, Tim Adams. "John Cacioppo: 'Loneliness Is Like an Iceberg- It Goes Deeper Than We Can See,'" *Guardian,* February 28, 2016; www.theguardian.com/science/2016/feb/28/loneliness-is-like-an-iceberg-john-cacioppo-social-neuroscience-interview

8. Valtorta NK, Kanaan M, Gilbody S, *et al.* "Loneliness and social isolation as risk factors for coronary heart disease and stroke: systematic review and meta-analysis of longitudinal observational studies." *Heart (*2016); **102:** 1009-1016; https://heart.bmj.com/content/102/13/1009

9. Barbara L. Fredrickson, Michael A. Cohn, Kimberly A. Coffey, Jolynn Pek, and Sandra M. Finkel, "Open Hearts Build Lives: Positive Emotions, Induced Through Loving-Kindness Meditation, Build Consequential Personal Resources," *Journal of Personality and Social Psychology 95,* no. 5 (2008): 1045-1062; www.ncbi.nlm.nih.gov/pmc/articles/PMC3156028/

10. "The Inflammatory Reflex: A New Understanding of Immunology," SetPoint Medical, https://setpointmedical.com/science/inflammatory-reflex/; Rediger, Jeffrey M.D. ('2020). *Cured: The Life-Changing Science Of Spontaneous Healing.* New York: Flatiron Books.

11. Bethany Kok and Barbara Fredrickson, "Upward Spirals of the Heart: Autonomic Flexibility, as Indexed by Vagal Tone, Reciprocally and Prospectively Predicts Positive Emotions and Social Connectedness," Biological *Psychology 85,* no. 3 (2010): 432-436; Rediger, Jeffrey M.D. (2020). *Cured: The Life-Changing Science Of Spontaneous Healing.* New York: Flatiron Books.

12. https://draxe.com/health/oxytocin/

13. W.W. Ishak, M. Kahloon, and H. Fakhry, "Oxytocin Role in Enhancing Well-Being: A Literature Review," *Journal of Affective Disorders* 130, nos. 1-2 (April 2011): 1-9; A. Steptoe, S. Dockray, and J. Wardle, "Positive Affect and Psychobiological Processes Relevant to Health," *Journal of Personality* 77, no. 6 (December 2009): 1747-76.

14. S. Dockray and A. Steptoe, "Positive Affect and Psychobiological Processes," *Neuroscience and Biobehavioral Reviews* 35, no. 1 (September 2010): 69-75; R. Ader, ed., *Psychoneuroimmunology,* 4th ed. (Burlington, MA: Elsevier Academic Press, 2011).

15. A. F. Chou et al., "Social Support and Survival in Young Women with Breast Carcinoma," *Psycho-oncology* 21, no. 2 (February 2012): 125-33.

16. K. L. Weihs et al., "Dependable Social Relationships Predict Overall Survival in Stages II and III Breast Carcinoma Patients." *Journal of Psychosomatic Research* 59, no. 5 (November 2005): 299-306; J. Holt-Lunstad, T. B. Smith, and J. B. Layton, "Social Relationships and Mortality Risk: A Meta-Analytic Review," *PLOS Medicine* 7, no. 7 (July 27, 2010): e1000316.

Section 2: Relationships Reflect Me: What Do You See?
Chapter 2: My Soul Deserves Peace

1. M. Gershon, (1998). "The Second Brain: The Scientific Basis of Gut Instinct and a Groundbreaking New Understanding of Nervous Disorders of the Stomach and Intestines," First Edition. New York: Harper.

2. "The Inflammatory Reflex: A New Understanding of Immunology," SetPoint Medical, https://setpointmedical.com/science/inflammatory-reflex/;
Rediger, Jeffrey M.D. (2020). *Cured: The Life-Changing Science Of Spontaneous Healing.* New York: Flatiron Books.

3. HeartMath Institute Research Staff, (2016). *Science of the Heart: Exploring the Role of the Heart in Human Performance. Volume 2;*
https://heartfirehealingllc.com/3-brains-head-heart-

gut/; *https://spinalresearch.com.au/three-brains-head-heart-gut-sometimes-conflict/*

4. Barbara L. Fredrickson, Michael A. Cohn, Kimberly A. Coffey, Jolynn Pek, and Sandra M. Finkel, "Open Hearts Build Lives: Positive Emotions, Induced Through Loving-Kindness Meditation, Build Consequential Personal Resources," *Journal of Personality and Social Psychology 95,* no. 5 (2008): 1045-1062; www.ncbi.nlm.nih.gov/pmc/articles/PMC3156028/; Rediger, Jeffrey M.D. (2020). *Cured: The Life-Changing Science Of Spontaneous Healing.* New York: Flatiron Books.

5. Grote V, Lackner H, Kelz C, Trapp M, Aichinger F, Puff H, Moser M, "Short-term effects of pulsed electromagnetic fields after physical exercise are dependent on autonomic tone before exposure." *Eur J Appl Physiol.* 2007 Nov; 101(4): 495-502. doi: 10.1007/s00421-007-0520-x. Epub 2007 Aug 3. PMID: 17674028; https://pubmed.ncbi.nlm.nih.gov/17674028/

6. Miller JG, Kahle S, Hastings PD. Roots and Benefits of Costly Giving: Children Who Are More Altruistic Have Greater Autonomic Flexibility and Less Family Wealth. Psychol Sci. 2015 Jul; 26(7): 1038-45. doi: 10.1177/0956797615578476. Epub 2015 May 26. PMID: 26015412; PMCID: PMC4504814; https://pubmed.ncbi.nlm.nih.gov/26015412/; Rediger, Jeffrey M.D. (2020). *Cured: The Life-Changing Science Of Spontaneous Healing.* New York: Flatiron Books.

7. Bethany Kok and Barbara Fredrickson, "Upward Spirals of the Heart: Autonomic Flexibility, as Indexed by Vagal Tone, Reciprocally and Prospectively Predicts Positive Emotions and Social Connectedness," Biological *Psychology 85,* no. 3 (2010): 432-436

8. Everett L. Worthington Jr. & Michael Scherer (2004) Forgiveness is an emotion-focused

coping strategy that can reduce health risks and promote health resilience: theory, review, and hypotheses, Psychology & Health, 19:3, 385-405, DOI: 10.1080/0887044042000196674; https://www.tandfonline.com/doi/abs/10.1080/08870440 42000196674

9. Porges, Stephen. (2004). Neuroception: A Subconscious System for Detecting Threats and Safety. ZERO TO THREE. 24; https://www.researchgate.net/publication/210294378_N euroception_A_Subconscious_System_for_Detecting_T hreats_and_Safety; Rediger, Jeffrey M.D. (2020). *Cured: The Life-Changing Science Of Spontaneous Healing.* New York: Flatiron Books. 10. Worthington, Everett L. "The Science of Forgiveness." Department of Psychology: Virginia Commonwealth University. (April 2020); https://www.templeton.org/wp-content/uploads/2020/06/Forgiveness_final.pdf; https://greatergood.berkeley.edu/article/item/the_new_sc ience_of_forgiveness/

Section 2: Relationships Reflect Me: What Do You See?
Chapter 3: Into Me You See

1. Firestone, R. W. 1985. *The Fantasy Bond: Structure of Psychological Defenses.* Santa Barbara, CA: The Glendon Association; Shapiro, D. 2000. *Dynamics of Character: Self-Regulation in Psychopathology.* New York: Basic Books.

2. Cozolino, L. 2006. *The Neuroscience of Human Relationships: Attachment and the Developing Social Brain.* New York: Norton; Schore, A. N. 1994. *Affect Regulation and the Origin of the Self: The Neurobiology of Emotional Development.* Hillsdale, NJ: Erlbaum; Schore, A. N. 2003a. *Affect Regulation and Disorders of the Self.* New York: Norton; Schore, A. N. 2009,

"Relational Trauma and the Developing Right Brain: An Interface of Psychoanalytic Self Psychology and Neuroscience." In *Self and Systems: Explorations in Contemporary Self-Psychology.* Annals of the New York Academy of Sciences, vol. 1159. Edited by W. J. Coburn and N. Van Der Heide. Boston: Blackwell; Siegal, D. J. 1999. *The Developing Mind: Toward a Neurobiology of Interpersonal Experience.* New York: Guilford Press; Siegal, D. J., and M. Hartzell. 2003. *Parenting from the Inside Out: How a Deeper Self-Understanding Can Help You Raise Children Who Thrive.* New York: Tarcher.

3. E. Z. Tronich, "Emotions and Emotional Communication in Infants," *American Psychologist 44,* no. 2 (1989): 112. See also E. Tronick, *The Neurobehavioral and Social-Emotional De3velopment of Infants and Children* (New York: W. W. Norton & Company, 2007); E. Tronick and M. Beeghly, "Infants' Meaning-Making and the Development of Mental Health Problems," *American Psychologist 66,* no. 2 (2011): 107; and A. V. Sravish, et. Al., "Dyadic Flexibility During Face-to-Face Sill-Face Paradigm: A Dynamic Systems Analysis of Its Temporal Organization," *Infant Behavior and Development 36,* no. 3 (2013): 432-37.

4. C. Trevarthen, "Musicality and the Intrinsic Motive Pulse: Evidence from Human Psychobiology and Rhythms, Musical Narrative, and the Origins of Human Communication," *Muisae Scientiae,* special issue, 1999, 157-213.

5. Ainsworth, M. D. S. 1989. "Attachments Beyond Infancy." *American Psychologist 44* (4): 709-16; Ainsworth, M. D. S., M. C. Blehar, E. Waters, and S. Wall. 1978. *Patterns of Attachment: A Psychological Study of the Strange Situation.* Hillsdale, NJ: Erlbaum; Bowlby, J. 1982. *Attachment and Loss.* Vol. 1,

Attachment (2nd ed.). New York: Basic Books; Bowlby, J. 1988. *A Secure Base: Parent-Child Attachment and Healthy Human Development.* New York: Basic Books; Main, M., and E. Hesse. 1990. "Parents' Unresolved Traumatic Experiences Are Related to Infant Disorganized Attachment Status: Is Frightened and/or Frightening Parental Behavior the Linking Mechanism?" In *Attachment in the Preschool Years: Theory, Research, and Intervention.* Edited by M. T. Greenberg, D. Cicchetti, and E. M. Cummings. Chicago: University of Chicago Press.

6. M. Main, "Overview of the Field of Attachment," *Journal of Consulting and Clinical Psychology 64,* no. 2 (1996): 237-43.

7. D. Finkelhor, R. K. Ormrod, and H. A. Turner, "Polyvictimization and Trauma in a National Longitudinal Cohort," *Development and Psychopathology 19,* no. 1 (2007): 149-66; J. D. Ford, et al., "Poly-victimization and Risk of Posttraumatic, Depressive, and Substance Use Disorders and Involvement in Delinquency in a National Sample of Adolescents," *Journal of Adolescent Health 46,* no. 6 (2010): 545-52; J. D. Ford, et al., "Clinical Significance of a Proposed Development Trauma Disorder Diagnosis: Results of an International Survey of Clinicians," *Journal of Clinical Psychiatry 74,* no. 8 (2013): 841-49.

8. Main, M. (1990). "Cross-cultural studies of attachment organization: Recent studies, changing methodologies, and the concept of conditional strategies." *Human Development,* 33, 48-61.

9. Main, M. (1990). "Cross-cultural studies of attachment organization: Recent studies, changing methodologies, and the concept of conditional strategies." *Human Development,* 33, 48-61; E. Hesse and M. Main, "Frightened, Threatening, and Dissociative Parental Behavior in Low-Risk Samples: Description,

Discussion, and Interpretations," *Development and Psychopathology 18,* no. 2 (2006): 309-43. See also E. Hesse and M. Main, "Disorganized Infant, Child, and Adult Attachment: Collapse in Behavioral and Attentional Strategies," *Journal of the American Psychoanalytic Association 48,* no. 4 (2000): 1097-127; M. Main, "Overview of the Field of Attachment," *Journal of Consulting and Clinical Psychology 64,* no. 2 (1996): 237-43.

10. S. D. Pollak, et al., "Recognizing Emotion in Faces: Developmental Effects of Child Abuse and Neglect," *Developmental Psychology 36,* no. 5 (2000): 679.

11. M. H. van Ijzendoorn, C. Schuengel, and M. Bakermans-Kranenburg, "Disorganized Attachment In Early Childhood: Meta-analysis of Precursors, Concomitants, and Sequelae," *Development and Psychopathology 11* (1999): 225-49.

12. R. Yehuda, et al., "Vulnerability to Posttraumatic Stress Disorder in Adult Offspring of Holocaust Survivors," *American Journal of Psychiatry 155,* no. 9 (1998): 1163-71. See also R. Yehuda, et al., "Relationship Between Posttraumatic Stress Disorder Characteristics of Holocaust Survivors and Their Adult Offspring," *American Journal of Psychiatry 155,* no. 6 (1998): 841-43; R. Yehuda, et al., "Parental Posttraumatic Stress Disorder as a Vulnerability Factor for Low Cortisol Trait in Offspring of Holocaust Survivors," *Archives of General Psychiatry 64,* no. 9 (2007): 1040 and R. Yehuda, et al., "Maternal, Not Paternal PTSD is Related to Increased Risk for PTSD in Offspring of Holocaust Survivors," *Journal of Psychiatric Research 42,* no. 13 (2008): 1104-11; R. Yehuda, et al., "Transgenerational Effects of PTSD in Babies of Mothers Exposed to the WTC Attacks during Pregnancy," *Journal of Clinical Endocrinology and Metabolism 90* (2005): 4115-18.

13. C. M. Chemtob, Y. Nomura, and R. A. Abramovitz, "Impact of Conjoined Exposure to the World Trade Center Attacks and to Other Traumatic Events on the Behavioral Problems of Preschool Children," *Archives of Pediatrics and Adolescent Medicine 162,* no. 2 (2008): 126. See also P. J. Landrigan, et al., "Impact of September 11 World Trade Center Disaster on Children and Pregnant Women," *Mount Sinai Journal of Medicine 75,* no. 2 (2008): 129-34.

14. G. Saxe, et al., "Relationship Between Acute Morphine and the Course of PTSD in Children with Burns," *Journal of the American Academy of Child & Adolescent Psychiatry 40,* no. 8 (2001): 915-21. See also G. N. Saxe, et al., "Pathways to PTSD, Part I: Children with Burns," *American Journal of Psychiatry 162,* no. 7 (2005): 1299-304.

15. N. W. Boris, M. Fueyo, and C. H. Zeanah, "The Clinical Assessment of Attachment in Children Under Five," *Journal of the American Academy of Child & Adolescent Psychiatry 36,* no. 2 (1997): 291-93; K. Lyons-Ruth, "Attachment Relationships Among Children with Aggressive Behavior Problems: The Role of Disorganized Early Attachment Patterns," *Journal of Consulting and Clinical Psychology 64,* no. 1 (1996), 64; Louise Hertsgaard, et al., "Adrenocortical Responses to the Strange Situation in Infants with Disorganized Attachment Relationships," *Child Development 66,* no. 4 (1995): 1100-6; Gottfried Spangler, and Klaus E. Grossmann, "Biobehavioral Organization in Securely and Insecurely Attached Infants," *Child Development 64,* no. 5 (1993): 1439-50.

16. Family Pathways Project, https://www.challiance.org/academics/research/family-studies-lab/family-pathways-project

17. K. Lyons-Ruth and D. Block, "The Disturbed Caregiving System: Relations Among Childhood

Trauma, Maternal Caregiving, and Infant Affect and Attachment," *Infant Mental Health Journal 17,* no. 3 (1996): 257-75.

18. K. Lyons-Ruth and D. Jacobvitz, "Attachment Disorganization: Genetic Factors, Parenting Contexts, and Developmental Transformation from Infancy to Adulthood," in *Handbook of Attachment: Theory, Research, and Clinical Applications,* 2nd ed., ed. J. Cassidy and R. Shaver (New York: Guilford Press, 2008), 666-97. See also E. O'Connor, et al., "Risks and Outcomes Associated with Disorganized/Controlling Patterns of Attachment at Age Three Years in the National Institute of Child Health & Human Development Study of Early Child Care and Youth Development," *Infant Mental Health Journal 32,* no. 4 (2011): 450-72; and K. Lyons-Ruth, et al., "Borderline Symptoms and Suicidality/Self-Injury."

19. M. H. van Ijzendoorn, C. Schuengel, and M. Bakermans-Kranenburg, "Disorganized Attachment in Early Childhood: Meta-Analysis of Precursors, Concomitants, and Sequelae, *Development and Psychopathology 11* (1999): 225-49.

20. E. Warner, et al., "Can the Body Change the Score? Application of Sensory Modulation Principles in the Treatment of Traumatized Adolescents in Residential Settings," *Journal of Family Violence 28,* no. 7 (2003): 729-38.

21. Mikulincer, Mario and Shaver, Phillip. "Attachment in Adulthood: Structure, Dynamics, and Change." (2007): New York: The Guilford Press; https://www.academia.edu/34596672/Attachment_in_A dulthood_Structure_Dynamics_and_Change_Mario_Mi kulincer_PhD_Phillip_R_Sha_pdf

Section 2: Relationships Reflect Me: What Do You See?
Chapter 4: Come Out of Hiding

1. Brown, Brene, Ph. D., LMSW. (2012). *Daring Greatly: How the Courage to Be Vulnerable Transforms the Way We Live, Love, Parent, and Lead.* New York: Avery.
2. Brown, Brene, Ph. D., LMSW. (2012). *Daring Greatly: How the Courage to Be Vulnerable Transforms the Way We Live, Love, Parent, and Lead.* New York: Avery.
3. Doidge, Norman M.D. (2007). *The Brain That Changes Itself.* New York: Penguin Books.
4. Lane, R. D., L. Ryan, L. Nadel, and L. Greenberg. 2015. "Memory Reconsolidation, Emotional Arousal, and the Process of Change in Psychotherapy: New Insights from Brain Science." *Behavioral and Brain Sciences 38:* 1-64.
5. Cozolino, L. (2006). *The Neuroscience of Human Relationships: Attachment and the Developing Social Brain.* New York: Norton.
6. Lickerman, A. (2012). *The Undefeated Mind: On the Science of Constructing an Indestructible Self.* Deerfield, FL: Health Communications.
7. Schore, A. N. 2003b. *Affect Regulation and the Repair of the Self.* New York: Norton; Welling, H. 2012. "Transformative Emotional Sequence: Towards a Common Principle of Change." *Journal of Psychotherapy Integration 22:* 109-36.

Section 2: Relationships Reflect Me: What Do You See?
Chapter 5: The Art of Developing True Intimacy

1. Kelly, Matthew. (2005). *The Seven Levels Of Intimacy: The Art Of Loving and the Joy of Being Loved.* Second Edition. New York: Beacon Publishing.

2. Kelly, Matthew. (2005). *The Seven Levels Of Intimacy: The Art Of Loving and the Joy of Being Loved.* Second Edition. New York: Beacon Publishing.

Section 3: Unraveling the Imprint of Trauma
Chapter 1: The Dream-Like State of Surviving Trauma & How to Move Past Surviving into Thriving

1. Van Der Kolk, Bessel M.D. (2014). *The Body Keeps The Score: Brain, Mind, And Body In The Healing Of Trauma.* New York: Penguin Books.
2. Rita Carter and Christopher D. Frith, *Mapping the Mind* (Berkeley: University of California Press, 1998). See also A. Bechara, et al., "Insensitivity to Future Consequences Following Damage to Human Prefrontal Cortex," *Cognition 50,* no. 1 (1994): 7-15; A. Pascual-Leone, et al., "The Role of the Dorsolateral Prefrontal Cortex in Implicit Procedural Learning," *Experimental Brain Research 107,* no. 3 (1996): 479-85; and S. C. Rao, G. Rainer, and E. K. Miller, "Integration of What and Where in the Primate Prefrontal Cortex," *Science 276,* no. 5313 (1997): 821-24.
3. H. S. Duggal, "New-Onset PTSD After Thalamic Infarct," *American Journal of Psychiatry 159,* no. 12 (2002): 2113-a. See also R. A. Lanius, et. Al., "Neural Correlates of Traumatic Memories in Posttraumatic Stress Disorder: A Functional MRI Investigation," *American Journal of Psychiatry 158,* no. 11 (2001): 1920-22; and I. Liberzon, et al., "Alteration of Corticothalamic Perfusion Ratios During a PTSD Flashback," *Depression and Anxiety 4,* no. 3 (1996): 146-50.
4. R. Noyes Jr. and R. Kletti, "Depersonalization in Response to Life-Threatening Danger," *Comprehensive Psychiatry 18,* no. 4 (1977): 375-84. See also M. Sierra, and G. E. Berrios, "Depersonalization: Neurobiological

Perspectives," *Biological Psychiatry 44,* no. 9 (1998): 898-908.

5. Van Der Kolk, Bessel M.D. (2014). *The Body Keeps The Score: Brain, Mind, And Body In The Healing Of Trauma.* New York: Penguin Books.

6. Ivan Pavlov, *Lectures on Conditioned Reflexes.* NY International Publishers, 1928.

7. Pavlov, I. P. (1927). *Conditioned Reflexes: An Investigation of the Physiological Activity of the Cerebral Cortex.* Translated and edited by Anrep, GV (Oxford University Press, London, 1927); http://psychclassics.yorku.ca/Pavlov/lecture6.htm

8. Van Der Kolk, Bessel M.D. (2014). *The Body Keeps The Score: Brain, Mind, And Body In The Healing Of Trauma.* New York: Penguin Books.

9. R. Noyes Jr. and R. Kletti, "Depersonalization in Response to Life-Threatening Danger," *Comprehensive Psychiatry 18,* no. 4 (1977): 375-84. See also M. Sierra, and G. E. Berrios, "Depersonalization: Neurobiological Perspectives," *Biological Psychiatry 44,* no. 9 (1998): 898-908.

10. Van Der Kolk, Bessel M.D. (2014). *The Body Keeps The Score: Brain, Mind, And Body In The Healing Of Trauma.* New York: Penguin Books.

11. R. Joseph, *The Right Brain and the Unconscious* (New York: Plenum Press, 1995).

12. Van Der Kolk, Bessel M.D. (2014). *The Body Keeps The Score: Brain, Mind, And Body In The Healing Of Trauma.* New York: Penguin Books.

13. Van Der Kolk, Bessel M.D. (2014). *The Body Keeps The Score: Brain, Mind, And Body In The Healing Of Trauma.* New York: Penguin Books.

14. B. Roozendaal, B. S. McEwen, and S. Chattarji, "Stress, Memory and the Amygdala," *Nature Reviews Neuroscience 10,* no. 6 (2009): 423-33.

Megan Van Zyl

Section 3: Unraveling the Imprint of Trauma
Chapter 2: Mindfulness: Ending the Phantom Existence

1. S. S. Tomkins, *Affect, Imagery, Consciousness* (vol. 1, *The Positive Affects)* (New York: Springer, 1962); S. S. Tomkins, *Affect, Imagery, Consciousness (*Vol. 2, *The Negative Affects) (*New York: Springer, 1963).
2. G. Rizzolatti and L. Craighero "The Mirror-Neuron System," *Annual Review of Neuroscience 27* (2004): 169-92. See also M. Iacoboni, et al., "Cortical Mechanisms of Human Imitation," *Science* 286, no. 5449 (1999): 2526-28; C. Keysers and V. Gazzola, "Social Neuroscience: Mirror Neurons Recorded in Humans," *Current Biology 20,* no. 8 (2010): R353-54; J. Decety and P. L. Jackson, "The Functional Architecture of Human Empathy," *Behavioral and Cognitive Neuroscience Reviews* 3 (2004): 71-100; M. B. Schippers, et al., "Mapping the Information Flow from One Brain to Another During Gestural Communication," *Proceedings of the National Academy of Sciences of the United States of America 107,* no. 20 (2010): 9388-93; and A. N. Meltzoff and J. Decety, "What Imitation Tells Us About Social Cognition: A Rapprochement Between Developmental Psychology and Cognitive Neuroscience," *Philosophical Transactions of the Royal Society, London 358* (2003): 491-500.
3. P. Ekman, *Emotions Revealed: Recognizing Faces and Feelings to Improve Communication and Emotional Life* (New York: Macmillan, 2007); P. Ekman, *The Face of Man: Expressions of Universal Emotions in a New Guinea Village* (New York: Garland STPM Press, 1980).
4. Van Der Kolk, Bessel M.D. (2014). *The Body Keeps The Score: Brain, Mind, And Body In The Healing Of Trauma.* New York: Penguin Books.

5. Van Der Kolk, Bessel M.D. (2014). *The Body Keeps The Score: Brain, Mind, And Body In The Healing Of Trauma.* New York: Penguin Books.
6. D. Diorio, V. Viau, and M. J. Meaney, "The Role of the Medial Prefrontal Cortex (Cingulate Gyrus) in the Regulation of Hypothalamic-Pituitary-Adrenal Responses to Stress," *Journal of Neuroscience* 13, no. 9 (September 1993): 3839-47; J. P. Mitchell, M. R. Banaji, and C. N. Macrae, "The Link Between Social Cognition and Self-Referential Thought in the Medial Prefrontal Cortex," *Journal of Cognitive Neuroscience* 17, no. 8 (2005): 1306-15.
7. B. A. van der Kolk, "Clinical Implications of Neuroscience Research in PTSD," *Annals of the New York Academy of Sciences* 1071 (2006): 277-93.
8. D. J. Siegel, *The Mindful Therapist: A Clinician's Guide to Mindsight and Neural Integration* (New York: W. W. Norton, 2010).
9. J. E. LeDoux, "Emotion Circuits in the Brain," *Annual Review of Neuroscience 23,* no. 1 (2000): 155-84.
10. S. W. Porges, "Stress and Parasympathetic Control," *Stress Science: Neuroendocrinology* 306 (2010). See also S. W. Porges, "Reciprocal Influences Between Body and Brain in the Perception and Expression of Affect," in *The Healing Power of Emotion: Affective Neuroscience, Development & Clinical Practice,* Norton Series on Interpersonal Neurobiology (New York: W. W. Norton, 2009), 27.
11. Van Der Kolk, Bessel M.D. (2014). *The Body Keeps The Score: Brain, Mind, And Body In The Healing Of Trauma.* New York: Penguin Books.
12. K. Kosten and F. Giller Jr., "Alexithymia as a Predictor of Treatment Response in Post-Traumatic Stress Disorder," *Journal of Traumatic Stress* 5, no. 4 (October 1992): 563-73.

13. R. D. Lane, et al., "Impaired Verbal and Nonverbal Emotion Recognition in Alexithymia," *Psychosomatic Medicine* 58, no. 3 (1996): 203-10.

14. Gendlin, Eugene. (1982). *Focusing.* New York: Random House Digital.

15. A. D'Argembeau, et al., "Distinct Regions of the Medial Prefrontal Cortex Are Associated with Self-Referential Processing and Perspective Taking," *Journal of Cognitive Neuroscience* 19, no. 6 (2007): 935-44. See also N. A. Farb, et al., "Attending to the Present: Mindfulness Meditation Reveals Distinct Neural Modes of Self-Reference," *Social Cognitive and Affective Neuroscience* 2, no. 4 (2007): 313-22; and B. K. Holzel, et al., "Investigation of Mindfulness Meditation Practitioners with Voxel-Based Morphometry," *Social Cognitive and Affective Neuroscience* 3, no. 1 (2008): 55-61.

16. C. Steuwe, et al., "Effect of Direct Eye Contact in PTSD Related to Interpersonal Trauma: An fMRI Study of Activation of an Innate Alarm System," *Social Cognitive and Affective Neuroscience* 9, no. 1 (January 2012): 88-97.

17. P. Schilder, "Depersonalization." In *Introduction to a Psychoanalytic Psychiatry* (New York: International Universities Press, 1952), p. 120.

18. D. A. Bakal, *Minding the Body: Clinical Uses of Somatic Awareness* (New York: Guilford Press, 2001); M. Cloitre, et al., "Posttraumatic Stress Disorder and Extent of Trauma Exposure as Correlates of Medical Problems and Perceived Health Among Women with Childhood Abuse," *Women & Health* 34, no. 3 (2001): 1-17; D. Lauterbach, R. Vora, and M. Rakow, "The Relationship Between Posttraumatic Stress Disorder and Self-Reported Health Problems," *Psychosomatic Medicine* 67, no. 6 (2005): 939-47.

Section 3: Unraveling the Imprint of Trauma
Chapter 3: Become a Curious Observer of Your Internal
World & Own Your Emotional Brain

1. R. L. Bluhm, et al., "Alterations in Default Network Connectivity in Posttraumatic Stress Disorder Related to Early-Life Trauma," *Journal of Psychiatry & Neuroscience 34,* no. 3 (2009): 187. See also J. K. Daniels, et al., "Switching Between Executive and Default Mode Networks in Posttraumatic Stress Disorder: Alterations in Functional Connectivity." *Journal of Psychiatry & Neuroscience 35,* no. 4 (2010): 258.

2. Van Der Kolk, Bessel M.D. (2014). *The Body Keeps The Score: Brain, Mind, And Body In The Healing Of Trauma.* New York: Penguin Books, pg. 212.

3. S. G. Hofmann, et al., "The Effects of Mindfulness-Based Therapy on Anxiety and Depression: A Meta-Analytic Review," *Journal of Consulting and Clinical Psychology* 78, no. 2 (2010): 169-83; J. D. Teasdale, et al., "Prevention of Relapse/Recurrence in Major Depression by Mindfulness-Based Cognitive Therapy," *Journal of Consulting and Clinical Psychology* 68 (2000): 615-23; L.E. Carlson, et al., "One Year Pre-Post Intervention Follow-up of Psychological, Immune, Endocrine and Blood Pressure Outcomes of Mindfulness-Based Stress Reduction (MBSR) in Breast and Prostate Cancer Outpatients," *Brain, Behavior, and Immunity 21,* no. 8 (2007): 1038-49.

4. B. K. Holzel, et al., "Stress Reduction Correlates with Structural Changes in the Amygdala," *Social Cognitive and Affective Neuroscience* 5 (2010): 11-17; B. K. Holzel, et al., "Mindfulness Practice Leads to Increases in Regional Brain Gray Matter Density," *Psychiatry Research* 191, no. 1 (2011): 36-43; A.D. Craig, "Interoception: The Sense of Physiological Condition of

the Body," *Current Opinion on Neurobiology* 13 (2003): 500-5.

5. V. Felitti, et al., "Relationship of Childhood Abuse and Household Dysfunction to Many of the Leading Causes of Death in Adults: The Adverse Childhood Experiences (ACE) Study," *American Journal of Preventive Medicine* 14, no. 4 (1998): 245-58.

6. A. A. Lima, et al., "The Impact of Tonic Immobility Reaction on the Prognosis of Post-traumatic Stress Disorder," *Journal of Psychiatric Research* 44, no. 4 (March 2010): 224-28; P. Janet, *L'automatisme psychologique* (Paris: Felix, Alcan, 1889).

7. Van Der Kolk, Bessel M.D. (2014). *The Body Keeps The Score: Brain, Mind, And Body In The Healing Of Trauma.* New York: Penguin Books.

8. S. F. Maier and M. E. Seligman, "Learned Helplessness: Theory and Evidence," *Journal of Experimental Psychology: General* 105, no. 1 (1976). 3. See also M. E. Seligman, S. F. Maier, and J. H. Geer, "Alleviation of Learned Helplessness in the Dog," *Journal of Abnormal Psychology 73,* no. 3 (1968): 256; and R. L. Jackson, J. H. Alexander, and S. F. Maier, "Learned Helplessness, Inactivity, and Associative Deficits: Effects of Inescapable Shock on Response Choice Escape Learning," *Journal of Experimental Psychology: Animal Behavior Processes 6,* no. 1 (1980): 1.

9. P. Ekman, R. W. Levenson, and W. V. Friesen, "Autonomic Nervous System Activity Distinguishes Between Emotions," *Science 221* (1983): 1208-10; J. H. Jackson, "Evolution and Dissolution of the Nervous System," in *Selected Writings of John Hughlings Jackson,* ed. J. Taylor (London: Stapes Press, 1958): 45-118.

10. J. Bowlby, *A Secure Base: Parent-Child Attachment and Healthy Human Development* (New York: Basic Books, 2008), 103.

11. K. L. Walsh, et al., "Resiliency Factors in the Relation Between Childhood Sexual Abuse and Adulthood Sexual Assault in College-Age Women," *Journal of Child Sexual Abuse 16,* no. 1 (2007): 1-17.
12. B. A. van der Kolk, J. C. Perry, and J. L. Herman, "Childhood Origins of Self-Destructive Behavior," *American Journal of Psychiatry* 148 (1991): 1665-71.
13. E. E. Nelson and J. Panksepp, "Brain Substrates of Infant-Mother Attachment: Contributions of Opioids, Oxytocin, and Norepinephrine," *Neuroscience & Biobehavioral Reviews 22,* no. 3 (1998): 437-52. See also J. Panksepp, et al., "Endogenous Opioids and Social Behavior," *Neuroscience & Biobehavioral Reviews 4,* no. 4 (1981): 473-87; and J. Panksepp, E. Nelson, and S. Siviy, "Brain Opioids and Mother-Infant Social Motivation," *Acta paediatrica 83,* no. 397 (1994): 40-46.
14. Van Der Kolk, Bessel M.D. (2014). *The Body Keeps The Score: Brain, Mind, And Body In The Healing Of Trauma.* New York: Penguin Books, pg. 146.
15. S. A. Strassels, "Economic Burden of Prescription Opioid Misuse and Abuse," *Journal of Managed Care Pharmacy 15,* no. 7 (2009): 556-62; C. B. Nemeroff, et al., "Differential Responses to Psychotherapy Versus Pharmacotherapy in Patients with Chronic Forms of Major Depression and Childhood Trauma," *Proceedings of the National Academy of Sciences of the United States of America 100,* no. 24 (2003): 14293-96. See also C. Heim, P.M. Plotsky, and C. B. Nermeroff, "Importance of Studying the Contributions of Early Adverse Experience to Neurobiological Findings in Depression," *Neuropsychopharmacology 29,* no. 4 (2004): 641-48.
16. B. E. Carlson, "Adolescent Observers of Martial Violence," *Journal of Family Violence 5,* no. 4 (1990): 285-99. See also B. E. Carlson, "Children's Observations of Interparental Violence," in *Battered*

Women and Their Families, ed. A. R. Roberts (New York: Springer, 1984), 147-67; J. L. Edleson, "Children's Witnessing of Adult Domestic Violence," *Journal of Interpersonal Violence 14,* no. 8 (1999): 839-70.

17. J. E. Stevens, "The Adverse Childhood Experiences Study- the Largest Public Health Study You Never Heard Of," *Huffington Post,* October 8, 2012, http://www.huffingtonpost.com/jane-ellen-stevens/the-adverse-childhood-exp_1_b_1943647.html

18. L. A. Sroufe and W. A. Collins, *The Development of the Person: The Minnesota Study of Risk and Adaptation from Birth to Adulthood* (New York: Guilford Press, 2009); and L. A. Sroufe, "Attachment and Development: A Prospective, Longitudinal Study from Birth to Adulthood," *Attachment & Human Development 7,* no. 4 (2005): 349-67.

19. D. Jacobvitz and L. A. Sroufe, "The Early Caregiver-Child Relationship and Attention-Deficit Disorder with Hyperactivity in Kindergarten: A Prospective Study," *Child Development 58,* no. 6 (December 1987): 1496-504.

20. G. H. Elder Jr., T. Van Nguyen, and A. Caspi, "Linking Family Hardship to Children's Lives," *Child Development 56,* no. 2 (April 1985): 361-75.

21. E. E. Werner and R. S. Smith, *Overcoming the Odds: High Risk Children from Birth to Adulthood* (Ithaca, NY, and London: Cornell University Press, 1992).

22. P. K. Trickett, J. G. Noll, and F. W. Putnam, "The Impact of Sexual Abuse on Female Development: Lessons from a Multigenerational, Longitudinal Research Study," *Development and Psychopathology 23* (2011): 453-76. See also J. G. Noll, P. K. Trickett, and F. W. Putnam, "A Prospective Investigation of the Impact of Childhood Sexual Abuse on the Development

of Sexuality," *Journal of Consulting and Clinical Psychology 71* (2003): 575-86.

23. Van Der Kolk, Bessel M.D. (2014). *The Body Keeps The Score: Brain, Mind, And Body In The Healing Of Trauma.* New York: Penguin Books.

24. A. A. T. S. Reinders, et al., "One Brain, Two Selves," *NeuroImage 20* (2003): 2119-25. See also E. R. S. Nijenhuis, O. Van der Hart, and K. Steele, "The Emerging Psychobiology of Trauma-Related Dissociation and Dissociative Disorders," in *Biological Psychiatry,* vol. 2., eds. H. A. H. D'Haenen, J. A. den Boer, and P. Wilner (West Sussex, UK: Wiley 2002), 1079-198; J. Parvizi and A. R. Damasio, "Consciousness and the Brain Stem," *Cognition 79* (2001): 135- 59.

25. P. Ogden, K. Minton, and C. Pain, *Trauma and the Body* (New York: Norton, 2010); P. Ogden and J. Fisher, *Sensorimotor Psychotherapy: Interventions for Trauma and Attachment* (New York: Norton, 2014).

26. P. Levine, *In an Unspoken Voice* (Berkeley, CA: north Atlantic Books); P. Levine, *Waking the Tiger* (Berkeley, CA: North Atlantic Books).

27. http://modelmugging.org/

Section 3: Unraveling the Imprint of Trauma
Chapter 4: Reversing the Amnesia of Trauma to Fully Integrate Your Brain

1. J. D. Payne, et al., "Sleep Increases False Recall of Semantically Related Words in the Desse-Roediger-McDermott Memory Task," *Sleep* 29 (2006): A373.

2. J. L. McGaugh and M. L. Hertz, *Memory Consolidation* (San Francisco: Albion Press, 1972); L. Cahill and J. L. McGaugh, "Mechanisms of Emotional Arousal and Lasting Declarative Memory," *Trends in Neurosciences* 21, no. 7 (1998): 294-99.

3. Y. D. Van Der Werf, et al. "Special Issue: Contributions of Thalamic Nuclei to Declarative Memory Functioning," *Cortex* 39 (2003): 1047-62. See also B. M. Elzinga and J. D. Bremner, "Are the Neural Substrates of Memory the Final Common Pathway in Posttraumatic Stress Disorder (PTSD)?" *Journal of Affective Disorders* 70 (2002): 1-17; L. M. Shin, et al., "A Functional Magnetic Resonance Imaging Study of Amygdala and Medial Prefrontal Cortex Responses to Overtly Presented Fearful Faces in Posttraumatic Stress Disorder," *Archives of General Psychiatry* 62 (2005): 273-81.

4. S. Freud, *Inhibitions Symptoms and Anxiety* (1914), 150. See also Strachey, *Standard Edition of the Complete Psychological Works.*

5. B. A. van der Kolk and R. Fisler, "Dissociation and the Fragmentary Nature of Traumatic Memories: Overview and Exploratory Study," *Journal of Traumatic Stress* 8 (1995): 505-25; J. W. Hopper and B. A. van der Kolk, "Retrieving, Assessing, and Classifying Traumatic Memories: A Preliminary Report on Three Case Studies of a New Standardized Method," *Journal of Aggression, Maltreatment & Trauma* 4 (2001): 33-71; J. J. Freyd and A. P. DePrince, eds., *Trauma and Cognitive Science* (Binghamton, NY: Haworth Press, 2001), 33-71.

6. E. F. Loftus, S. Polonsky, and M. T. Fullilove, "Memories of Childhood Sexual Abuse: Remembering and Repressing," *Psychology of Women Quarterly* 18, no. 1 (1994): 67-84. L. M. Williams, "Recall of Childhood Trauma: A Prospective Study of Women's Memories of Child Sexual Abuse," *Journal of Consulting and Clinical Psychology* 62, no. 6 (1994): 1167-76.

7. L. M. Williams, "Recovered Memories of Abuse in Women with Documented Child Sexual Victimization

Histories," *Journal of Traumatic Stress* 8, no. 4 (1995): 649-73.

8. J. Panksepp and L. Biven, *The Archaeology of Mind: Neuroevolutionary Origins of Human Emotions,* Norton Series on Interpersonal Neurobiology (New York: W. W. Norton, 2012).

9. J. D. Bremner, "Does Stress Damage the Brain?" *Biological Psychiatry* 45, no. 7 (1999): 797-805; I. Liberzon, et al., "Brain Activation in PTSD in Response to Trauma-Related Stimuli," *Biological Psychiatry* 45, no. 7 (1999): 817-26; L. M. Shin, et al., "Visual Imagery and Perception in Posttraumatic Stress Disorder: A Positron Emission Tomographic Investigation," *Archives of General Psychiatry* 54, no. 3 (1997): 233-41; L. M. Shin, et al., "Regional Cerebral Blood Flow During Script-Driven Imagery in Childhood Sexual Abuse0 Related PTSD: A PET Investigation," *American Journal of Psychiatry* 156, no. 4 (1999): 575-84.

10. Van Der Kolk, Bessel M.D. (2014). *The Body Keeps The Score: Brain, Mind, And Body In The Healing Of Trauma.* New York: Penguin Books.

11. J. W. Pennebaker, *Opening Up: The Healing Power of Expressing Emotions* (New York: Guilford Press, 2012), 12-19.

12. J. W. Pennebaker, *Opening Up: The Healing Power of Expressing Emotions* (New York: Guilford Press, 2012), 12-50.

13. A. M. Krantz, and J. W. Pennebaker, "Expressive Dance, Writing, Trauma, and Health: When Words Have a Body," *Whole Person Healthcare* 3 (2007): 201-29.

14. B. Van der Kolk, et al., "A Randomized Clinical Trial of EMDR, Fluoxetine and Pill Placebo in the Treatment of PTSD: Treatment Effects and Long-Term Maintenance," *Journal of Clinical Psychiatry* 68 (2007): 37-46.

15. R. Greenwald, "Eye Movement Desensitization and Reprocessing (EMDR): A New Kind of Dreamwork?" *Dreaming* 5, no.1 (1995): 51-55. R. Cartwright, et al., "REM Sleep Reduction, Mood Regulation and Remission in Untreated Depression," *Psychiatry Research* 121, no. 2 (2003): 159-67. R. Cartwright, et al., "Role of REM Sleep and Dream Affect in Overnight Mood Regulation: A Study of Normal Volunteers," *Psychiatry Research* 81, no. 1 (1998): 1-8.

16. R. Greenberg, C. A. Pearlman, and D. Gampel, "War Neuroses and the Adaptive Function of REM Sleep," *British Journal of Medical Psychology* 45, no. 1 (1972): 27-33. B. van der Kolk, et al., "Nightmares and Trauma: A Comparison of Nightmares After Combat with Lifelong Nightmares in Veterans," *American Journal of Psychiatry* 141, no. 2 (1984): 187-90.

17. R. Stickgold, et al., "Sleep-Induced Changes in Associative Memory," *Journal of Cognitive Neuroscience* 11, no. 2 (1999): 182-93. R. Stickgold, "Of Sleep, Memories and Trauma," *Nature Neuroscience* 10, no. 5 (2007): 540-42; and B. Rasch, et al., "Odor Cues During Slow-Wave Sleep Prompt Declarative Memory Consolidation," *Science* 315, no. 5817 (2007): 1426-29.

18. E. J. Wamsley, et al., "Dreaming of a Learning Task Is Associated with Enhanced Sleep-Dependent Memory Consolidation," *Current Biology* 20, no. 9 (May 11, 2010): 850-55.

19. R. Stickgold, "EMDR: A Putative Neurobiological Mechanism of Action," *Journal of Clinical Psychology* 58 (2002): 61-75.

20. B. A. van der Kolk, et al., "A Randomized Clinical Trial of Eye Movement Desensitization and Reprocessing (EMDR), Fluoxetine, and Pill Placebo in the Treatment of Posttraumatic Stress Disorder: Treatment Effects and

Long-Term Maintenance," *Journal of Clinical Psychiatry* 68, no. 1 (2007): 37-46.

21. A. Freud and D. T. Burlingham, *War and Children* (New York: New York University Press, 1943).

22. Van Der Kolk, Bessel M.D. (2014). *The Body Keeps The Score: Brain, Mind, And Body In The Healing Of Trauma.* New York: Penguin Books.

23. Moshe Szyf, Patrick McGowan, and Michael J. Meaney, "The Social Environment and the Epigenome," *Environmental and Molecular Mutagenesis* 49, no. 1 (2008): 46-60. D. Mehta et al., "Childhood Maltreatment Is Associated with Distinct Genomic and Epigenetic Profiles in Posttraumatic Stress Disorder," *Proceedings of the National Academy of Sciences of the United States of America* 110, no. 20 (2013): 8302-7.

24. A. J. Bennett, et al., "Early Experience and Serotonin Transporter Gene Variation Interact to Influence Primate CNS Function," *Molecular Psychiatry* 7, no. 1 (2002): 118-22. C. S. Barr, et al., "Interaction Between Serotonin Transporter Gene Variation and Rearing Condition in Alcohol Preference and Consumption in Female Primates," *Archives of General Psychiatry* 61, no. 11 (2004): 1146.

25. E. Warner, et al., "Can the Body Change the Score? Application of Sensory Modulation Principles in the Treatment of Traumatized Adolescents in Residential Settings," *Journal of Family Violence* 28, no. 7 (2013): 729-38. Van Der Kolk, Bessel M.D. (2014). *The Body Keeps The Score: Brain, Mind, And Body In The Healing Of Trauma.* New York: Penguin Books.

Section 3: Unraveling the Imprint of Trauma
Chapter 5: Healing the Abandoned Heart

1. Van Der Kolk, Bessel M.D. (2014). *The Body Keeps The Score: Brain, Mind, And Body In The Healing Of Trauma.* New York: Penguin Books.
2. Van Der Kolk, Bessel M.D. (2014). *The Body Keeps The Score: Brain, Mind, And Body In The Healing Of Trauma.* New York: Penguin Books.
3. McFarlane, Alexander. (2000). "Posttraumatic stress disorder: A model of the longitudinal course and the role of risk factors." *The Journal of clinical psychiatry* 61 Suppl 5. 15-20; discussion 21. Van Der Kolk, Bessel M.D. (2014). *The Body Keeps The Score: Brain, Mind, And Body In The Healing Of Trauma.* New York: Penguin Books.
4. J. N. Demos, *Getting Started with Neurofeedback* (New York: W. W. Norton, 2005). R. J. Davidson, "Affective Style and Affective Disorders: Prospectives from Affective Neuroscience," *Cognition and Emotion* 12, no. 3 (1998): 307-30; R. J. Davidson, et al., "Regional Brain Function, Emotion and Disorders of Emotion," *Current Opinion in Neurobiology* 9 (1999): 228-34.
5. M. Arns, et al., "Efficacy of Neurofeedback Treatment in ADHD: The Effects on Inattention, Impulsivity and Hyperactivity: A Meta-Analysis," *Clinical EEG and Neuroscience* 40, no. 3 (2009): 180-89; T. Rossiter, "The Effectiveness of Neurofeedback and Stimulant Drugs in Treating AD/HD: Part I: Review of Methodological Issues," *Applied Psychophysiology and Biofeedback* 29, no. 2 (June 2004): 95-112; T. Rossiter, "The Effectiveness of Neurofeedback and Stimulant Drugs in Treating AD/HD: Part II: Replication," *Applied Psychophysiology and Biofeedback* 29, no. 4 (2004): 233-43.

6. R. J. Castillo, "Culture, Trance, and the Mind-Brain, "*Anthropology of Consciousness* 6, no. 1 (March 1995): 17-34. B. Inglis, *Trance: A Natural History of Altered States of Mind* (London: Paladin, 1990).

7. E. G. Peniston and P. J. Kulkosky, "Alpha-Theta Brainwave Neuro-Feedback Therapy for Vietnam Veterans with Combat-Related Post-traumatic Stress Disorder," *Medical Psychotherapy* 4 (1991): 47-60.

8. E. G. Peniston and P. J. Kulkosky, "Alpha-Theta Brainwave Neuro-Feedback Therapy for Vietnam Veterans with Combat-Related Post-traumatic Stress Disorder," *Medical Psychotherapy* 4 (1991): 47-60.

9. R. C. Kessler, "Posttraumatic Stress Disorder: The Burden to the Individual and to Society," *Journal of Clinical Psychiatry* 61, suppl. 5 (2000): 4-14. R. Acicerno, et al., "Risk Factors for Rape, Physical Assault, and Posttraumatic Stress Disorder in Women: Examination of Differential Multivariate Relationships," *Journal of Anxiety Disorders* 13, no. 6 (1999): 541-63; H. D. Chilcoat and N. Breslau, "Investigations of Causal Pathways Between PTSD and Drug Use Disorders," *Addictive Behaviors* 23, no. 6 (1998): 827-40.

10. E. G. Peniston, "EMG Biofeedback-Assisted Desensitization Treatment for Vietnam Combat Veterans Post-traumatic Stress Disorder," *Clinical Biofeedback and Health* 9 (1986): 35-41. Eugene G. Peniston and Paul J. Kulkosky," Alpha-Theta Brainwave Neurofeedback for Vietnam Veterans with Combat-Related Post-Traumatic Stress Disorder," *Medical Psychotherapy* 4, no. 1 (1991): 47-60.

11. P. Healy, "The Anguish of War for Today's Soldiers, Explored by Sophocies," *New York Times,* November 11, 2009. http://www.outsidethewirellc.com/projects/theater-of-war/overview

12. Van Der Kolk, Bessel M.D. (2014). *The Body Keeps The Score: Brain, Mind, And Body In The Healing Of Trauma*. New York: Penguin Books. http://www.urbanimprov.org/ http://www.traumacenter.org/initiatives/psychosocial.php http://the-possibility-project.org/ http://www.shakespeare.org/education/for-youth/shakespeare-courts/

Section 4: Wakefulness
Chapter 1: Wake up to Spiritual Reality

1. Frankl, Viktor; Eds. Batthyány, Alexander; Tallon, Andrew. (2010). *The Feeling of Meaninglessness: A Challenge to Psychotherapy and Philosophy*. Milwaukee: Marquette University Press; ISBN: 978-0874627589.
2. Frankl, Victor. (1959-2007). *Man's Search For Meaning: An Introduction to Logotherapy*. Boston: Beacon Press; ISBN 0-8070-1426-5.
3. Thomas, Dr. Caroline Bedell. "John Hopkins Precursors Study," John Hopkins University Medical School. 1948 until now; http://noetichealth.com/DissertationE-book.pdf; http://www.epi.umn.edu/cvdepi/study-synopsis/johns-hopkins-precursors-study/; https://pages.jh.edu/jhumag/0601web/study.html
4. Gail Ironson et al., "An Increase in Religiousness/Spirituality Occurs after HIV Diagnosis and Predicts Slower Disease Progression over Four Years in People with HIV," *Journal of General Internal Medicine* 21 (2006): 62-68. Church, Dawson. (2008). *The Genie in Your Genes*. Fulton, CA: Energy Psychology Press. Pg. 65.
5. Eric R. Kandel, *In Search of Memory: The Emergence of a New Science of Mind* (New York: Norton, 2006). Leaf,

Caroline. (2013). *Switch On Your Brain.* Grand Rapids, Michigan: BakerBooks. Pg. 55-56.

6. Leaf, Caroline. (2013). *Switch On Your Brain.* Grand Rapids, Michigan: BakerBooks. Pg. 35. Glen Rein and Rollin McCraty, "Local and Nonlocal Effects of Coherent Heart Frequencies on Conformational Changes of DNA," Proceedings of the Joint USPA/IAPR Psychotronics Conference, Milwaukee, Wisconsin, 1993, http://www.heartmath.org/templates/ihm/e-newsletter/publication/2012/winter/emotions-can-change-your-dna.php; Rollin McCraty et al., "Modulation of DNA Conformation By Heart-Focused Intention." HeartMath Research Center, Institute of HeartMath, publications no. 03-08, Boulder Creek, CA, 2003.

Section 4: Wakefulness
Chapter 2: We all Have an Incurable Disease

1. https://www.newyorker.com/books/page-turner/our-strange-unsettled-history-of-mourning
2. https://onlinelibrary.wiley.com/doi/full/10.1002/pon.3067; https://www.latimes.com/archives/la-xpm-1989-05-11-mn-3291-story.html
3. Yale University. "Negative beliefs about aging predict Alzheimer's disease in study." ScienceDaily. ScienceDaily, 7 December 2015. <www.sciencedaily.com/releases/2015/12/151207145906.htm>.
4. https://news.yale.edu/2002/07/29/thinking-positively-about-aging-extends-life-more-exercise-and-not-smoking
5. Meador C K. Hex death: voodoo magic or persuasion? *South Med J* 1992; 85; 244–247.
6. Reeves RR, Ladner ME, Hart RH, Burke RS. Nocebo effects with antidepressant clinical drug trial

placebos. *Gen Hosp Psychiatry* 2007;29:275–277. doi: 10.1016/j.genhosppsych.2007.01.010

7. Moseley JB, Wrap NP, O'Malley K. "Arthroscopic Surgery for Osteoarthritis of the Knee (letter)." *New England Journal of Medicine.* 2 (347): 1718-1719.

8. https://pharmaceutical-journal.com/article/feature/nocebo-the-placebo-effects-evil-twin#fn_5

9. https://bronnieware.com/blog/regrets-of-the-dying/

Made in the USA
Columbia, SC
27 January 2023

10882108R00198